W9-BNA-111

ALZHEIMER'S WIDOW

ALZHEIMER'S WIDOW

by Marilyn Strothers

To my children Carla and Letha,
to Dr. Thomas Miller and Dr. Lee Harris who held
my hand all the way,
and to my husband, Warren, where it all began.

ACKNOWLEDGEMENTS

WITH GRATEFUL APPRECIATION I acknowledge every individual who encouraged me to write this book. I would list every name but there were so many I do not remember all of them.

Dottie Rose-Brennan was the first to read part of the manuscript and said that I had a message that should be told.

I cannot adequately express my thanks to Janet Byrne. After reading the entire manuscript she was a veritable bank of encouragement while still offering an honest appraisal of the book's strengths and weaknesses.

Unsolicited financial support was received from many friends. I thank them for anticipating that I might need such support.

Triple hugs of appreciation are bestowed on my children who came to my aid, often by long-distance telephone, when my lack of computer technology overwhelmed me.

I am also very grateful for use of the following:
Where Do I Begin (Love Theme)
Words by Carl Sigman
Music by Francis Lai
Copyright © 1970, 1971 by Famous Music Corporation
Copyright Renewed 1998, 1999 and Assigned to Famous Music Corporation and Major Songs Company
All Rights for the World excluding the U.S.A. Controlled and Administered by Famous Music Corporation
International Copyright Secured   All Rights Reserved

PROLOGUE

I AM A WIDOW. In church I do not sit with the group of women who sit in the same pew because they have become widowed by the death of their spouse. There are about eight or ten of them now sitting together. It is an eerie sight. I've often wondered if the women who are not yet widows wonder as I do how long it will be before we join the others.

But I am a widow as surely as they are, although my husband lives, and breathes, and keeps doctors appointments, and pushes the grocery cart, and sleeps beside me every night.

I have properly classified myself, based on a lexicographer's definition of "Widow: "A woman who has lost her husband by death." That part of the definition excludes me, but there is a part of the definition, "to deprive of something greatly loved and needed," that allows me to be included in the status.

It is not with deprecation that I refer to the pew where the widows sit as Widows' Row. I knew their husbands, visited them with their illnesses of cancer, heart disease, or whatever the cause of their suffering was. And when death came, I attended the funeral of the deceased and hugged and grieved with their loved ones.

The disease that has made me a widow by robbing me of "the thing I loved and needed" is none of the above. It is Alzheimer's disease. Maybe you have never heard of it. Maybe you have heard of it but it has not affected you or anyone close to you. It does not count that Great Aunt Tillie who lives in California, while you live in Maine has it. Both the distance in relationship to Aunt Tillie, and the distance in miles that separate you prevent the knowledge of the horror of the disease from emerging to you as a reality. That is why I am sharing my experience, in case you ever need to know, although my sincere hope is that you never do.

If I have enemies, I do not know them. However, I suspect that along the sojourn of life I have encountered individuals that, for whatever reason, may dislike me. Whether they be my enemy, or merely someone who does not care for me personally, I would forgive either case before wishing upon them the heartache, pain, and suffering of having a loved one become afflicted with Alzheimer's dementia.

Alzheimer's is an insidious neurological disease deriving its name from the German neurologist who identified it in 1906. It is unlike other diseases in that both the afflicted person and the caregiver suffer dissimilarly but equally. So intertwined is the affect of the Alzheimer's sufferer and his (or her) caregiver that books are written about the patient but for the caregiver.

My story is for the caregiver who may or may not have been alerted by a family doctor or neurologist to expect changes in behavior to occur in the loved one who has been diagnosed to have Alzheimer's dementia. The changes will be in the form of mood swings, bouts of depression, agitation, anxiety, and a variety of other idiosyncratic behaviors that the caregiver will never before have known to be characteristic of their loved one.

Through the pages of this book, I invite the caregiver to walk with me inside of those general headings and actually see the downed head that cannot be gently prodded, persuaded by argument, or patiently coaxed into looking up from its heavy darkness.

Where do I begin? The words merely question how to begin telling a story that many people need to know about. They rode into my consciousness on the tune to which they were sung in the Paramount motion picture, "Love Story". The sad, haunting tune became embedded in my mind, pervading all further thoughts on the narrative.

Part of the story is told in the form of journal entries. For many years I have maintained journals, entering daily such insignificant items as whether the sky was blue or gray, when the first ants appeared in summer, whether it rained or snowed, or whether my husband and I had a meeting of minds sexually. Little did I know that by putting to paper these inconsequential details I would unwittingly record warning signs of the horrific fate that would befall my husband, our children, and me.

All facts in the narrative are true. Dialogue, except where indicated otherwise, is between my husband and me, so personal pronouns are often used, although given names were used when recorded in the journal. Pseudonyms for all characters are used throughout the story, however they represent real people with whom we have interacted.

The name I have chosen to use as my husband's is Job, as in the biblical character who endured much suffering yet never wavered in faith to his God. It is the perfect name for my husband. The biblical Job had seven sons and three daughters. One of the trials that befell him was that all of his children died. Eventually he became the father of other children.

My Job and I had a son that died in infancy. We now have two daughters who have been and are a blessing in our lives. The older one is Carol. This fictitious name was chosen for her because in French it means, "song of joy." The English meaning is, "strong and womanly." Both meanings fit her well.

Amy is the name I will call our younger daughter. It means "sweet, and well-loved." This name is easily applicable to our youngest child but could have been given to either child had not each of our children deserved to have her own name.

ONE

❦

ONCE, THERE WAS A WONDERFULLY GOOD PART of my husband's and my life together. Presented first is the part that has become almost intolerable for me to bear. The good parts, where there was only love and happiness, emerge as the story unfolds. That is more preferable to me than the reverse order. The changes that have come about in our lives are not the fault of either of us, but of the dread Alzheimer's disease.

After the fact, after changes in your loved one have become so acute that professional help must be sought, after the diagnosis and you start receiving written materials on the disease, you realize that the warning signs that all was not well were there all along. But they went unrecognized as an oncoming irreversible mental decline.

The signals began for us at least two years before an actual diagnosis was made. I noticed them in Job's driving. I had for some time thought he took curves too fast. He was never able to convince me that driving faster when rounding curves made the car hold to the road better. When he would drive in this manner, sometimes I would complain about it. Usually, I did not.

Had it not been for a gift received at his retirement party (1989), the first sign of impending trouble may have escaped my notice.

Job loves classical music, and a co-worker knowing of his interest gave him a retirement gift of a pair of tickets to a Philadelphia Orchestra concert. We used those tickets and enjoyed the excitement of attending live concerts so much that we subscribed to tickets to attend all performances of the season. On our way to one concert we came to a busy intersection where the traffic signal was red. Job stopped briefly to obey the signal, but proceeded to go before the light turned to green. Only my warning of his oversight kept him from continuing through the red signal.

We traveled this route often to go to concerts or to visit relatives in the city. Job's habit of partially ignoring traffic signals caused me to become tense whenever we approached them. While he would usually pause briefly at red lights, he was not so diligent in observing Stop signs and would zip right through them without stopping at all. I began to feel so uncomfortable riding with him that I would only accompany him if I were the driver. A journal entry tells of my concern.

December 3, 1995 (Sunday)
    I had planned to attend church in the city but didn't feel up to it. We were going to the Academy of Music to hear "Messiah". I didn't feel up to doing that either, but we did go. Amy and James went with us. I did the driving. After the concert we had dinner at Marabella's. I had slept through most of the concert, imagine! For an entrée at dinner I only had soup. James and Amy went home to Maryland from the city, so that just left Job to drive us home. That gives you an idea of just how sick I was.

OFTEN JOB WOULD MENTION to me that as he was riding in his car, he would sometimes not recognize streets that he had traveled many times before. Not every incidence of these occurrences is recorded. There were times also when he would stop in the middle of a task he was about and just sit quietly doing nothing. I would ask why, and, never varying his answer, he would remark that he felt faint and that his stomach felt queasy.

January 14, 1996 (Sunday)
    I had planned to attend church with Job today, but he didn't go. He was up and dressed for church and went into the kitchen and ate a bowl of cereal. I was surprised when he came back into the bedroom and sat down. I had to ask him if he had changed his mind about going to church. He said he felt faint and his stomach felt queasy.

March 16, 1996
    Job didn't go to Sunday school or church. Complained of faintness and a queasy stomach.

May 24, 1996 (Friday)
    The morning is cool. I am sitting in our bedroom, as is Job. He is reading the paper. We've been up since 7:00, and it is 10:30 now. Job has been to the store and bought tomato, pepper, and flower plants. He had hoped to get them planted today, but he may not be able to. He was on the phone making reservations for our flight to Atlanta when he suddenly didn't feel well. I had to finish the transaction. Again, he complained of feeling faint and his stomach felt "queasy."

July 12, 1996 (Friday)
    My short-term memory is getting almost as bad as Job's. Time was I could miss a day of writing in my journal but could think backward to what happened on days missed. I find that I am not able to do that anymore.

July 27, 1996 (Saturday)
    Job forgot that today is Saturday and the fitness center opens later. He left the house at 6:05. The Center doesn't open until 7:00 today. Oh, well, he will only have about forty-five minutes to wait around.

September 17, 1996 (Tuesday)
    Job did some typing on the word processor all afternoon. Tonight he is supposed to go to Church Council meeting, but he isn't going. He doesn't feel up to it.

November 18, 1996 (Sunday)
    I had planned to attend church today. Job went to Sunday school. I was just about to run my bath water and get dressed when the telephone rang. When I answered, it was Pastor Shulz calling to tell me that Job wasn't feeling well. I went right away to bring him home. When I arrived at the church Job was lying on a little cot very near where the class was in session. I brought him home. Later in the day, he had two more spells of feeling faint.

THREE SPELLS OF FAINTNESS in one day caused me great concern, so I called our doctor. He prescribed medication that to me seemed more for indigestion than a remedy for someone suffering from a feeling of faintness. Even though, after taking the medication Job seems okay, I know that all is not well. When we've been to the doctor for his regular heart check-ups we have called these recurring spells to the doctor, but he cannot determine any cause for them. What will I do when he doesn't recover from one of these incidents?

TWO

January 5, 1997 (Sunday)

I was partially dressed for church and was enjoying a cup of coffee and a bagel as breakfast when the telephone rang. What now, I thought. Sure enough, it was not good news. Job wasn't feeling well again, and Grace Sands was calling to see if someone should bring him home, or would I come and pick him up. I thought the latter arrangement best, so I finished my coffee and bagel and set out.

When I arrived at church Job was lying on the same cot as before, only this time he was uncovered. He seemed nervous, jumpy, and talked incessantly. He wasn't sure if he had been scheduled to be an usher today. At home, at one time he began to breathe really heavily. He slept for a long time. When he awoke around 3:00, he went into the kitchen and finished eating the breakfast he had left before leaving for Sunday school.

January 22, 1997 (Wednesday)

Job was confused again about what day it is. I thought so when I heard him up so early. He seems not to be able to keep up with the days of the week and asks me time and again what day it is. I've suggested that he make himself a personal calendar and check the days off at day's end. He refuses to do that, although at one time he did. When he realized that it was not the day that we exercise at the gym, he crawled back into bed.

January 24, 1997 (Friday)

Job had an appointment with our family doctor for a check-up. He still drives himself to wherever he wants to go, but I went along with him today specifically to ask the doctor if he feels it is safe for Job to drive, since he has those periods of feeling faint. I was surprised that Dr. Miles thought it okay for Job to continue driving, but he said he was reluctant to take that privilege away. After all, he reasoned that if Job felt faint he could always pull off the road. I didn't tell him that Job always drives in the left lane. Always, unless he intends to make a right-hand turn.

February 3, 1997 (Monday)
Washed clothes. Dark ones. Job was at his "Ministry." I put the garbage out. Today it is quite warm, 10 degrees above normal. Onion grass is growing. Daffodils are still shooting up. My thoughts are so different from what they used to be. They are all in the here and now, all in the present moment. I hardly reflect on the past. I dare not think of the future. I know what's in store for me! There is no intimacy between Job and me. There's just day come. Day go. Night come. Night, fly away before I have had time to rest. Still, I watch his movements—standing at the dresser, patting the back pockets of his trousers to see that he has a clean handkerchief in each of them. That has been a daily ritual for all the years of our marriage. I watch him standing before the mirror tying his tie, and I am moved emotionally by his movements. I never let him see me watching. He looks so handsome in his clothes, without them though, he would never be chosen as a sculptor's model. His steps are purposeful. He never shuffles along. Age has caused his pace to be slower than it once was. He spends a lot of time standing at his dresser looking (flicking through) a zillion pieces of paper, old bills already paid but still in the envelopes they were mailed in, letters that he has not decided how to answer. When he turns to do something else he sometimes hesitates, not knowing I suppose exactly what thing he wants to do next.

February 9, 1997 (Sunday)
How blue the sky was today! Bright sunshine reflected off the virgin snow. Donnie shoveled out our driveway. Job cleaned ice and snow from one car. We were going to church, but when Job came inside after clearing snow from the car he said he felt light-headed, so I went to church alone.

June 1, 1997 (Sunday)

Welcome, June, although I'm only partly glad to see you. You've brought a wonderfully beautiful day, but you've also brought the halfway point of the year. It is hot when you're in the sun, but there's no humidity, so it's very comfortable. Job was usher in church today. I think it is the first time I've noticed how frail he is beginning to look.

June 20, 1997 (Friday)

The grandfather clock's wound. The cryptogram is done. I've eaten breakfast—cantaloupe, sticky bun, coffee, no bacon. Job went to the luncheon that Mellon Bank gives its retirees each year. I've cooked dinner. Job won't be hungry when he comes home. The luncheons are usually an all-day affair. Alone, I have too much time to think. Not focused thoughts. Scattered ones. Thoughts not of past things, nor future ones, except what is beyond life. I don't feel worried or unworried. I just think. Will Job get to a stage where I cannot care for him at home? Will I need to go into a nursing home? I've told the girls that I don't ever want to be a burden to them, and they should just put me in one. Now, I don't know. I don't even know if I want to get old.

July 14, 1997 (Monday)

This is how the day began: It has been quite hot and humid today. Of course the media made a meal off it, acting as if there has never during the existence of the planet earth been other hot, humid days. Did the usual Monday chores—washed, cleaned, etc. Job has been saying for days that he needs to send in money to the IRS because he has taken money from his IRA. On Saturday I told him that I would call the IRS, since he said he did not understand how to fill out the forms that he has requested they send him so that he can pay the rest of the money that he should send to avoid paying a penalty.

I wrote out a list of questions that we should ask when we call. I asked Job who the custodian of his IRA was. At first he seemed not to hear me, or not to understand what I was talking about. He was quiet for such a long time I had to ask my question again. This time, he burst into tears and cried, and cried, and cried. He said he didn't know what he was doing and that it was very frustrating to be that way. I told him that I would help with whatever problem he was having understanding about what should be done. He finally got himself together. He said he wasn't blaming me for anything. He knew I was only trying to help.

We got things squared away. I went to the store and bought file folders and labeled things. I know now that I must accompany him on all business transactions. The incident was very upsetting to me. A knot fixed itself in my stomach. I was close to tears. Oh, Time! What you do to us.

In the evening we went to Rita's for a water ice. I heard cicadas sing. This is the first time this year that I've heard their chorus.

July 26, 1997 (Saturday)

Job, as usual, went to the fitness center so that he would be there when it opened. I went later, but in time to do all of my time on each piece of equipment and still get home in time to leave for the family reunion (my side) in Teaneck, NJ between 10:30 and 11:00 AM. That's the time that we agreed on last night. I wrote the time and place of where we were going, and for what purpose, on a piece of cardboard and left it at the place Job had laid out to have breakfast. I told him I was leaving it there so that he would not have to ask me many, many times what time I wanted to leave, and where we were going. The note was propped up so that he could not miss seeing it. He had left the fitness center a full hour before I did, time enough to have prepared his breakfast, eaten it, and cleaned up the kitchen.

It was already 10:00 when I got home. He was sitting, unshaven, not dressed for going any place, and reading the newspaper. I made no move to wash the dishes, so he did them. It was after 12:00 when we finally got underway. It didn't really matter to me what time we arrived at the reunion, but I was angry, and he knew it.

On our way to the reunion he insisted that I disregard directions to the hotel that were sent by the reunion committee. Had I done so we would have gotten off at the wrong exit. I didn't listen to him and we arrived at the Marriott without incident.

August 17, 1997 (Sunday)

Early in the morning Job seemed restless. I wasn't sure if he was well or sick. I think it was his restlessness that awakened me just before 6:00. I tried to fall asleep again, as I still felt sleepy and tired. I looked over at him surreptitiously. I could only see one eye. It was open and darting about the way it does when he is confused or disoriented. I guessed that he was trying to figure out what day it was. He kept tossing and turning, this way and that way, occasionally moaning or sighing. By way of checking on his physical (and mental) health, I asked if he had taken his morning medication. He hadn't, got up and took it, and got back into bed.

I finally got up and went out to get the paper. When I laid it on the bed, he smiled and said it was a mighty big paper. Thinking that he was not aware of the day of the week, I told him that Sunday papers are always big.

When it is freshly mowed, our yard is beautiful, and it looks very large. Black-eyed Susans have flowered and are dying. Near the bank where the garden used to be, a few daylilies still are in bloom. It is 7:25 and already the sun is setting. The neighborhood, except for Donnie's dog, is quiet. Sometimes I feel like any moment I will break out and cry.

August 19, 1997 (Tuesday)

Job is at a church committee meeting, but I guess he will be home soon. It is 9:00. They have been meeting for 2 hours. It has been a heavenly day. At times it felt more like fall than August. Of course, there was fitness center to be gotten out of the way. After that Job went to the supermarket and food shopped. I cut a limb from one of the lilac bushes. It was a large limb. For a while I thought I wouldn't get it down. I had to do it while Job was out. If he were home he would pout by looking pitiful as I sawed away on it. But it needed to come down. I wish Job would come in from his meeting.

September 3, 1997 (Wednesday)

I almost wrote the date as August, but August what? There's nothing left of that month. Sometime between night and morn-ing it rained, taking away the humidity and overcast sky of yesterday. Today, in the early morning, some clouds remain, but when I looked out of the back window I saw a big swatch of clear blue. And by the time I got my wash on the line the sky had become a barrel of clear, blue water. Wind is up enough to knock small branches from our silver maple tree. I've tried several times to relax on the patio, but each time yellow jackets have driven me in. They are mean this time of year. It is as if they know they've got only a short time left to live. It feels like fall. It no longer looks like August. It looks like all past Septembers that I have known.

Job had asked me to carry a paper to Vera and Lance Bowman's house. It contained something about church business that he wanted them to have. I talked with them for a short while and was surprised when Vera mentioned that Job had told them that sometimes he gets so disoriented when driving that he must pull off the road to try to get himself together.

September 10, 1997 (Wednesday)

When I awoke this morning Job was lying in bed in a way that made me think he was not feeling well. Sure enough, when I asked if anything was wrong he said he had a nervous stomach. He said he had been up but had not felt up to taking his usual Wednesday shower. I brought him a basin of water and he washed himself. I put his toothbrush out, too, but he went into the bathroom to brush his teeth. I prepared his breakfast and carried it so that he could eat it in the bedroom. That is also where he ate lunch and dinner.

Late in the evening, quite by accident, I discovered the cause of his "illness". He was anxious about something that had happened at the church elder's meeting last night. Jane Adams, without realizing that she was doing so, told me something that Job probably did not want me to know. She said another Elder had accused Job of slighting a suggestion that he had made in favor of one made by another church member. I knew that Job would not intentionally have done that. At the time I did not associate the incident with the memory problem that I knew Job had. I became angry and told Job to call his pastor and talk with him about it. He did, and I thought the matter was settled.

September 11, 1997 (Thursday)

It is a dreary day. It rained last night and has off and on all day today. Job didn't go to the fitness center. He seems unnerved. My guess is that it is because of the elder thing. He did cook dinner for me, though, while I went to the hairdresser. He has an appointment to talk with Pastor tomorrow.

September 28, 1997 (Sunday)

It is a bit chilly today. It wasn't bad when I left for church (Job had gone to Sunday school). I didn't even wear a jacket. The sky is overcast. As the day wore on it became cooler, the clouds became darker and blotted out the little sunlight that had broken through. Job was the Elder of the day. This was to be his big moment. He would be in charge of a worship service and act like the Pastor that he had always wanted to be. He had spent a lot of time preparing for the duty of leading the service, but he came up woefully short of what I knew to be his expectations.

He looked so handsome in his brown suit and white shirt with lavender stripes. His hair, once mildly brown but all white now, shone beautifully. But he was pathetic in the way he was unable to keep abreast of what should come next. He read the Old Testament lesson and the Epistle, so it was time for the Gospel, but he announced the Epistle again. I was in our usual pew, third row from the front. Gary Larson was sitting right in front of me. I said loudly enough for Job to hear that it was the Gospel that was wanted here. When it was time for the Apostles' Creed, he got lost again. Wouldn't you think one of the other elders would just have begun saying it? But that isn't the Lutheran way, I guess. I looked back at Brian Adams and he did begin the Creed. The congregation joined in.

When it was time for the Lord's Prayer, Job was lost again and the organist called down from the choir loft to help him out.

OUR NEIGHBOR HAS PUT A JACK-O-LANTERN IN HIS WINDOW. The reflection from the electric candle that lights it makes a yellow/orange glow in the dark night. I like looking at it from my front window. Early this morning I was sweeping crabapples from our driveway. The same neighbor's children were playing on their front lawn, making children noises, playing children things, like climbing the big shade tree in their yard. When has that ever happened on this part of our street? Never, that I can remember. It was a welcome sight. Front lawns must always be carefully manicured in this small, suburban town. Swing sets and swimming pools in backyards are where children play.

October 7, 1997 (Tuesday)
    Why do I feel so sad? So like I will break down and weep, or scream? Job started out for the fitness center early again. He left home at 5:00 but realized his error and came back and left again later. Lately, he spends a lot of time on the word processor doing his church work. We don't communicate very much. Green leaves are beginning to turn to their fall colors. The neighborhood is quiet. No one calls. I do not call anyone.

October 8, 1997 (Wednesday)
    What a long strange year this has been! Everything seems so different. Job goes his own way, and I go mine, although last night there was a meeting of minds. Still, he is very stubborn, and just when I would be happy, enjoy being with him, he does something to make me really angry. Is it because we are getting old? At sixty-nine, I don't feel old. Is it because we've been married for such a long time? The forty years we've spent together has not seemed long to me. Oh, well.
    To make myself feel better I drove out to the mall and bought a couple of items. On the way home I drove out Kenas Road, riding along to the symphony of leaves in their fall colors. I drank in the visual music. All day it has been beautiful. Once home, I took a trip to the back of our yard and picked up apples from our trees that are producing prolifically this year.

October 16, 1997 (Thursday)
    After yesterday's rain, today is clear. The highlight of my day was my trip to the hairdresser. Other than that, just little things, catching up on things around the house left undone during our trip. Tonight, Job went to Elders' meeting. He wasn't gone long before he was home again. No one showed up for the meeting, he said. I always felt that that church did not appreciate all the things he did, and at this time of pastor vacancy, I am sure of it.

He says he is unaffected, but I know that he is. Then again, maybe he just got the meeting day mixed up. He gets a lot of things mixed up these days, and he won't accept anything I propose that might help him. For instance, I've asked him to keep a personal calendar so that he can keep track of the days of the week. I made a form for him to use when he answers the telephone. Who's calling—blank line for response, this is what we talked about—blank lines for responses—telephone number of the person calling—blank lines for responses. He refuses to use the forms.

October 18, 1997 (Saturday)

Rained again last night and was still cloudy today. Job was up early and dressed in his workout clothes for going to the fitness center, but he didn't go. His stomach felt queasy, and he said he felt dizzy. It's the church thing I guess. I had an errand to do for Job. Then I planned to go down to the city. First, I stopped by home to check on Job. He seemed okay, so I went on my way. When I got home hours later, he said he hadn't done anything or gone anywhere. His eyes looked teary, but he didn't seem sad.

October 29, 1997 (Wednesday)

Job went food shopping and afterwards sat in the living room reading the book that Carol had given him about the brain. He is having headaches periodically that I worry about. I hope he doesn't have a stroke or brain tumor.

December 4, 1997 (Thursday)

I'm not getting things done as quickly as I'd like. Went to the fitness center early and did all pieces of equipment for the full time. With time to spare before going to play the piano at the nursery school in Wrightstown, I ate breakfast. As soon as I finished playing the piano for the kids, and after they went off to their "work", I came home. Job was not at home. At church, I guess. He came home eventually but I didn't see much of him all afternoon. He sat in the living room. I napped in our bedroom. Today has been dreary. Last night it rained. I lay awake listening to it falling softly to the ground. It is 9:00. Job is at church. He has been there since 7:00. Especially during this time that the church is "calling" a pastor, I feel like a church widow. Job seems to be at church for one reason or another more often than he is at home.

THREE

March 2, 1998 (Tuesday)

The sun came out today. Job went to his ministry, which seems to be dwindling away. I know that he is hurt about it. It wasn't even 11:30 when I stopped by the church to tell him (I knew he planned to stop at the store) to buy eggs. As I parked and opened the car door, he was coming out of the door that leads up to the Pastor's office. I didn't learn until late evening that he had left earlier than he usually would have because he was unable to work on the computer that he uses. Seems the new Pastor (thank God they finally got one) is very computer knowledgeable, whereas the old pastor was not computer literate. Job did not know that a new system had been installed that he was not familiar with. I was angry that he was not told of the change. I felt very sorry for Job. I told him we must get him interested in another kind of ministry.

March 15, 1998 (Sunday)

Church again today. Job was the Elder. He is forgetting the Communion routine. He forgot to service Pastor, but Pastor tactfully reminded him of the oversight. Maybe no one else noticed. I hope not.

March 24, 1998 (Tuesday)

Job turned seventy-one today. His steps, once so springy, are getting slower. Little things frustrate him. How far he has gone downhill since I first met him as a twenty-five-year-old young man! I'm positively afraid to ride in the car with him. I've been telling him for the longest time that he drives too close to the curb. He reminds me that it was he who taught me to drive. Even when he came home one day with the outside mirror on the passenger side of the car knocked off he said something flew up from the street and knocked it off. I didn't for a minute believe it. I especially doubted his story when a short time later, as I was driving on the highway close to our house, I noticed that a speed sign had been bent backward a bit.

Pastor Shulz invited Job to go to a church circuit meeting. I'm glad. We had no other plans, so that was a good outing for him.

March 30, 1998 (Monday)

I am so angry with Job. We went to the senior citizen center and had our income tax prepared by one of the volunteers who does that service for center members. Mr. Banks assembled the completed tax forms. That is, he fastened with a paper clip those that should be mailed to IRS, and the ones to be filed with the State. He did the same for copies to be kept for our files. When we got home, Job took them apart and got them all mixed up. So today I have to go to Mr. Banks' home and ask him to straighten them out for me.

I feel so weepy. Maybe it's because Amy's wedding is coming up. Maybe it's because my sister Wilma is so sick and is trying so hard to get well. Maybe it's because I continue to worry about Job. He is just so different from how he used to be.

April 9, 1998 (Thursday)

Today is Maunday Thursday. There will be a church service tonight. Ordinarily, Job would have gone to the service. It was raining, and the wind was blowing pretty fiercely at the time he would have gone. Still, I've never known those conditions to keep him from going to a church service. He has worked hard all day. Maybe he is just tired. I didn't remind him of the service, and he went to bed. Always, I hope there will be some overture of intimacy, but he just puts his one arm around me as he has always done and says he loves me, adding "still". So, tonight he fell asleep. Oh, well, at seventy-one, he's allowed.

April 11, 1998 (Saturday)

Blossoms on our crabapple trees are fully open. In fact, petals

are already falling away, onto our cars, and onto the ground, making them look as if a light snow has fallen. It is a beautiful, cloudless day. Bright sunshine abounds. Daffodils are blooming, also
grape hyacinths. It is warm but not enough to be without a wrap.

May 11, 1998 (Monday)
    We went food shopping today. At night Job went to Elders'
meeting. When he came home he told me that he had asked the
Board to relieve him of his duties because of his memory problems. I think that was the wise thing to do. I know that he is
unhappy about having had to make the decision. That makes me
unhappy too.

May 31, 1998 (Sunday)
    Good-bye, May. You brought flowers that you usually bring,
and some that should have waited until June. It is not your fault
that time rushes on. Our yard is beautiful. Three different colors
of peonies bloomed: white, magenta, and lavender. Roses are out,
flags also.
    I went to Sunday school today but didn't stay for church.
When I got home I noticed that hollyhocks have started to open.
Yesterday and today have been warm, 90 degrees. Finally, the
handyman rotor-tilled our garden patch, and Job has set out
tomato plants. Birds sing cheerfully. Job is in the living room
reading the newspaper. He won't remember anything that he has
read. His mind is very bad. It was once such a good mind. I am
writing thank you notes to children who gave me gifts when the
nursery school closed last Thursday.

June 7, 1998 (Sunday)
    For the summer, morning service is at 9:30. Today was
Confirmation Sunday. Two children whom I had taught in Third
Grade Sunday school class, and another youngster that I didn't
know, were confirmed. Job was weepy in church. He often cries.
Sometimes I know the reason why, sometimes I don't. Today I
didn't know the reason.

June 9, 1998 (Tuesday)
    Is it spring or fall? It is hard to tell if you rely on the weath-

er as a barometer. For a while today there was sunshine and warmth. By afternoon, full-fledged clouds, dark blue in color, had set in, shutting out the sun, and making it positively cold. Dr. Miles called and wants me to have another blood test in three weeks. Job is at a church meeting tonight. Although he has resigned his post, the Elders have asked him to stay on as Elder Emeritus, at least until the end of the year. I guess that's considerate of them.

June 12, 1998 (Friday)

I almost forgot to wind the grandfather clock. Marty and I went to Wrightstown and quilted on the quilt she and the nursery school mothers are making for Amy's wedding. When I got home Job was playing a CD of Handel's "Messiah". He plays it a lot around Christmas and Easter but rarely at this time of year. I sat down and listened with him. In listening, I could see Thanksgivings and Christmases past, see myself going to the store to buy gifts for Job and the kids, see cold weather coming, see the children coming home to visit us during those holidays. I should play that CD more often, only I don't know how to work the stereo. I've always relied on Job to read directions and know how to operate things like stereos.

June 13, 1998 (Saturday)

We both went to the fitness center together. How I hate going, especially on Saturdays. June has not looked like June since it arrived. There's been no blue sky. Sometimes the sun comes out for part of the day but doesn't produce the blue, blue, June sky. Job played "Messiah" again. This time we listened to the old version, where the overture is played very slowly, and where William Warfield is the baritone.

June 14, 1998 (Sunday)

I feel so sad, so disconnected from the past, and dreading the future. I worry a lot about Job. My stomach gets in a knot. His mind, or rather his memory, is so bad. Sometimes I think he is simply faking forgetfulness. At other times I'm convinced that he is not faking and that causes me even greater concern. What is it heading toward? I guess I don't really want to know.

The grandfather clock is wound. I've had another busy, hectic day, which got off to a late start, because I stayed in bed until 7:30. Job ate breakfast and went up to the church and picked up newsletter material and carried it to the post office for mailing. He carried with him a refund check from our state income tax. The check was for twenty-four dollars, but when I checked the bank receipt the deposit showed thirty-four dollars. Turns out the teller had made the error.

When we got home from the bank, I insisted that Job look at the notice that had come from one of his IRA's. It has lain on his dresser for over two weeks with a note from me that we should discuss what should be done about it. He got very confused and dug out his other IRA that he also had questions about. I told him that I thought we should go to our local bank and let them help us answer whatever questions he had. He agreed to do that, but once in the bank, neither the teller nor I could help him understand what was to be done. Again, back at home he got angry with me, threw the papers on the bed, and went out and cut the grass. Luckily, I (of all people) understood what was to be done, so I made proper disposition of the matter, made notes accordingly, and filed the papers away.

He is very difficult to deal with. Anyway, the yard looks beautiful. Daylilies on the bank are blooming among all the weeds that the Township should have, but have not cut.

June 22, 1998 (Monday)
It has been cloudy all day but only spitting rain has resulted. Did my laundry. Trimmed a forsythia bush, bathed and dressed but didn't go out all day, just bummed around. I did call the custodian of one of Job's IRA's to be sure we had handled things correctly on the questionnaire they had sent us. Job didn't go to his church ministry today. He worked in the vegetable garden for a while, came inside, showered, dressed, and relaxed. This is what I've wanted him to do for the nine years we've been retired. Now, we have time and money to do interesting things but he is not in condition for enjoying it.

June 29, 1998 (Monday)
Job went to his ministry. I was surprised. He hasn't been for

a long time, two weeks, maybe. Our white lilies are fading. June, coming to a close.

July 13, 1998 (Monday)
   I like Mondays, even though they do seem "blue". I washed only one load of laundry. The house was tidied by 9:30. I left for Marty's and quilted until noon. Job didn't go to his ministry until 10:00. He got home well after I did but said he hadn't accomplished much. He said things get too confusing. I think he doesn't really want to be bothered anymore but doesn't know how to quit gracefully. I wonder if his bloodshot eye is getting better. It has hung around for two weeks, longer than ever before. Yesterday he had an incident of feeling faint while he was preparing his breakfast. He went into the living room and sat down. Amy happened to be visiting with us this weekend. She finished preparing his breakfast. Sometimes I catch him with a far-away look. He looks so sad. I wonder what he is thinking.

July 17, 1998 (Friday)
   This is the weekend that we can use the bed and breakfast get-away that Amy gave us as a Christmas gift. We are going to visit St. Michael Island, Maryland. We arrived at our destination around 4:00 Job had only worn a polo shirt with no T-shirt underneath. I suggested that he freshen up a bit before we went to dinner. This upset him, but I knew that for my benefit, and for other guests around us, he needed to freshen himself up with a sponge bath. I lay on the bed ignoring him and feigning sleep. Finally, I heard his favorite comment of late to himself: "I don't believe it." I knew immediately that the comment meant that he hadn't packed any underwear. I couldn't believe it either, as I had heard him opening and zipping up again and again the several compartments of his garment bag, as well as opening and closing the drawers of his dresser. I continued feigning sleep. When I "awoke", he told me what had happened. I didn't make an issue of it. We went to a store and bought as many as we needed to get us through our weekend vacation.

July 20, 1998 (Monday)
   We were up early. Job didn't go to his "ministry". I think he

has pretty much given it up, but I am not sure. He is very vague in his answers to anything I ask him. The weather is so hot, especially at night. Tonight Job went to elders' meeting. Brian Adams picked him up. I've told Brian that I am uneasy when he is out at night in the car. I'm afraid he might not remember the way home.

July 21, 1998 (Tuesday)
   Woke up early and couldn't get back to sleep, so I got up at 5:30. I didn't go outside much today. Job did a bit of gardening then came inside and said he was going over to the church for a little while. He came home maybe three hours later. That's okay. Once, I resented his spending so much time there. Now, I just hope it means that he is getting his confidence back.

August 9, 1998 (Sunday)
   Today, Betty (my niece) turned 70. A month and a few days from now, I'll catch up with her. When I went out to pick up the paper from the driveway it was still dark. There was some light, but light of night ending, not light of day beginning. Everything was so quiet, Daylight came fully as I sat drinking my morning cup of coffee and reading the newspaper. After church we visited Margie (our sister-in-law). She had prepared dinner for us. Job had called to tell her that we were coming for a visit.
   August has lost its July look and looks like August. The sky is not as blue. Today there were dark, blue/gray clouds. When our children were in grade school, this is the kind of day that signaled back-to-school-shoe-buying-time. I hope it rains soon. The ground is very dry. Our grass is brown, and flowers look wilted.

August 10, 1998 (Monday)
   I didn't have any housework to do except press a few pieces. It's a good thing. I was up fairly early, brought the paper in, sat down and had breakfast, not much; coffee, melon, toast, and juice. I knew Job was up. I saw him go into the bathroom, but he didn't come out to the kitchen to make his breakfast. When I went into the bedroom he was dressed but was lying on the bed. I brought him juice. He said he felt that juice was all his stomach could tolerate. Later, I gave him a piece of melon. For lunch

I gave him quartered tomato and four unsalted crackers.

It is quite humid. I tried to sweep crabapples from the drive-way. I hadn't been out any time at all before a yellow jacket went up my long, African, dress and stung me twice.

Job spent most of the day in our bedroom, sometime lying down, sometime sitting in his recliner. He doesn't look good, especially about the eyes. I've been watching them for over a month. He's quiet. Doesn't say anything unless I say something to him, and then he mostly mumbles answers.

I put the air conditioning on, although he said he didn't need it. He started to have a strange look, at one point looking as if he were trying to speak but couldn't. I ran and got a nitroglycerin tablet for him to put under his tongue. He seemed to feel better. He says the condition of dizziness and queasy stomach is the same as he has previously experienced, and he is sure it will eventually pass away.

I am waiting for Carol to call and say whether or not she is pregnant. Job is sitting in his recliner. The News Hour with Jim Lehrer is on, but Job is not watching as closely as he usually does. I feel anxious about something. Wilma's death is less than a month passed. Maybe that's it. But, I am also really worried about Job. I'm afraid I'm losing him.

FOUR

August 11, 1998 (Tuesday)

Job felt well enough to go to the fitness center. He was going alone but I advised against it and it is a good thing I did! We entered the center. Job was ahead of me. Immediately when he got to the box where charts are kept, he turned around but remained motionless, his arms still in the position of holding the chart. His eyes had a fixed stare. I rushed to him and asked what was the matter, but he didn't answer. I caught his arm. It felt rigid and cold. I asked again if he was okay. I think he said no, or else he started to say something unintelligible, as he has infrequently done before. There were chairs less than two feet away from where we were standing, but I didn't trust him to walk that far without falling down. I brought a chair to him. Brad Jensen, the head technician, saw there was trouble and came over to investigate what it was. We both tried to convince Job to go home. Finally we did, but not before Job protested that he was able to go on with his workout regimen.

I called our doctor as soon as we got home and described what had happened. He said I should bring Job to the office. I think the doctor suspected what was going on, because he sent us to the emergency room of the hospital. There was a certain neurologist with a private practice that he wanted us to see, but he knew that it might take weeks before we could see him. We were in the emergency room of the hospital from about 10:30 in the morning until 4:30 in the afternoon. By the time we drove the twenty minutes that it takes to get from the hospital to our home, what had happened from the time we got up at 5:30 in the morning, to the present, no longer was, and would never again be, a part of Job's memory.

We left the emergency room with two pages of printed information that included among other things the treatment he had received while there. The instructions read as follows:

> After leaving (the hospital), you should follow the instructions below.
> You were treated today by A. Turner Hickman, M.D. for: DEMENTIA, DELIRIUM. You were seen today for your confusion. You may not be able to remember things that have happened. You may have had hallucinations (seeing things that are not really there), been afraid or irritable. There are many causes for this condition. This may be short-term or long-term depending on the cause.

There were other general instructions, such as seeing his doctor regularly, take medicines as prescribed, avoid driving or operating machinery, etc. There was one specific instruction: Job was to call as soon as possible to be seen by a neurologist (whom they named), within 3 days for re-evaluation.

* * *

THIS DAY WAS TO BE THE TURNING POINT IN OUR LIVES, but we did not yet know it, and would not for months and years to come have a fuller understanding of how our lives would be changed. Even after we had kept our appointment with the neurologist, we remained naive as to what was to come.

FIVE

August 12, 1998 (Wednesday)
    It has been a lovely summer day. I describe it as shimmering loveliness. The day has been absolutely humidity free. It is the kind of day that I look out across our backyard and say how wonderful it is to be alive. This morning, pondering his condition, Job wept. Inside, where the tears were not visible, I wept as well. I tried to reassure him that I loved him and will always take care of him. We went to the supermarket. When we had almost completed our shopping, Job didn't feel well. I found a place for him to sit down on one of the shelves stocked with food items for sale. I went to the children's romper room and borrowed a chair for him to sit down in. After I had finished shopping, Job came to the cash register and paid for the groceries. Of things that occurred in his life years and years ago, Job's memory is perfect. But of things that happen from day to day, or for that matter, from moment to moment, he remembers practically nothing.

August 13, 1998 (Thursday)
    It is only Thursday but it feels like Friday. What a long year this has been, wearing out the century. Death clearing away people no longer needed. Babies being born as replacements. Carol called to confirm that she is pregnant. The baby is due February 19. Imagine that, our first grandchild.
    We kept our appointment with the neurologist. He gave Job a series of tests, then consulted with us. Job was to stop driving. I asked the doctor if Job could continue to drive the tractor lawnmower and he said, yes, if he had driven it before. What an unset-

tling turn of events this news is. We must accept that what we had thought to be a mere problem with Job's memory could well be early stage Alzheimer's dementia. In case it turns out after further tests that it is in fact Alzheimer's, the neurologist prescribed medicine that may retard progression of the disease, but we were informed that the disease can never be reversed, and there is no known cure for it. We scheduled an appointment to return to the neurologist for further tests. Further tests should determine if the cause of Job's memory trouble is the result of mini-strokes that he may have suffered.

Today at least there were no spells of faintness or queasy stomach.

How does a person who has been diagnosed with cancer feel? Pretty devastated I would think. What are the thoughts of his or her loved ones? At one of my class reunions, 35th, I think, I learned that a classmate, on learning that she had cancer, went into her basement and hanged herself.

We left the doctor's office with not that feeling of devastation. After all, the doctor had said that Job had done well in the tests he had already taken.

On our way home from the doctor's office we stopped at the drugstore and each of us picked out our own card to send to Amy for her birthday.

Calling the doctor's attention to any little ailment that he noticed was something Job has always done. I had often chided him for doing so. Until he was restricted from driving, he had always driven himself to keep doctor's appointments, so I don't know when he told the doctor of his forgetfulness. But at some point Dr. Miles gave the letter that follows to me. I do not recall when or why.

April 26, 1996

Craig J. Miles, M.D.
43 Grant Street
Holland, PA 19040

Re: Job Winters

Dear Craig:

I had the pleasure of seeing your patient, Job Winters for a neurologic consultation on April 26, 1996. Mr. Winters is a 69-year-old man who is referred for evaluation of forgetfulness.

Mr. Winters believes he has been having mild difficulties with his memory for about the past six months and is not aware that they are getting any worse. For example, he has trouble recalling people's names and, while in conversation, he can remember the person he is talking about and all their attributes but cannot come up with their name. If he is out driving, he may suddenly feel as if the area is unfamiliar and cannot recall how to get to where he is going, although within a few minutes it all comes back to him and he is able to get it together and has not been lost. On occasion, he will be walking into his basement to get something and when he gets there, he realizes he forgot what he was down there for and has to go back and start over again.

Despite the above complaints, the patient has not forgotten any significant events and continues to handle the finances at home without any errors. His wife is aware of the problems he has been having and does not think there is necessarily anything wrong.

Examination revealed Mr. Winters to be an alert and attentive, generally healthy appearing man with normal speech and language. He scored 27 out of 30 on the Mini-Mental State Examination. He was fully oriented to exact day and date and scored perfectly on serial 7's. However, he could only recall one out of three memory test objects in three minutes...

Impression: The neurologic examination was essentially within normal limits. The patient scored 27 out of 30 on the Mini-Mental State Examination, which is probably within the normal range for age...

I discussed with Mr. Winters the uncertainty regarding the cause of his forgetfulness. One possibility is cer-

tainly benign forgetfulness of aging which may simply be
a bit exaggerated in his case. Another possibility is very
early Alzheimer's disease, although there is certainly no
way to diagnose that nor am I suspicious for that at this
time. There is a significant family history of cerebrovas-
cular disease and, again, checking the CAT scan will be
important is this regard...

If the above studies prove negative, I don't believe any
further work-up is indicated at this time, although I
would like to see Mr. Winters back for a neurologic fol-
low-up in about six months to see if there has been any
further progression of symptoms. I have asked him to call
sooner as needed....

Yours sincerely,
Len

* * *

WHEN DID WE COME into possession of that letter? Where had it
been that I did not associate Job's increasing forgetfulness with the
possibility that he might have Alzheimer's? And how did I happen to come upon it now? To all the questions, my answer is, "I
do not know." But even had I looked at it every day, since I knew
nothing of the nature of the disease, I would not have known to
dread its coming. After all, Job has survived by-pass heart surgery,
several subsequent heart "incidents," a hernia operation, and surgery to remove a cancerous prostate. Could Alzheimer's disease be
more life threatening, or cause more disruption to our lives?

* * *

August 16, 1998 (Sunday)
We spent the weekend with Amy and James. Lois (my sister)
rode down to Maryland with us. Traffic wasn't bad going or coming. We had a lovely weekend with the newly married couple.
They are doing just fine. For the most part Job was alert and con-
tributed appropriately to conversations.

August 17, 1998 (Monday)
Job is quiet again and not remembering anything for more

than a few seconds. I tried to interest him in doing something but he showed no interest in doing anything that I suggested. Once he mentioned sending out letters to volunteers who will be recognized on "volunteer Sunday." I know that the church officers, and I suspect the pastor, do not want letters sent, but I offered no comment to him about sending them.

I wonder how we will make out at the fitness center tomorrow.

August, 18, 1998 (Tuesday)

Fitness center went just fine. Job did not do the full time on each piece of equipment, but he did workout on each piece that he is scheduled to do. As I expected, news on the television in the center was of President Clinton and Monica Lewinsky. It was talked about on the Jim Lehrer News Hour.

Since Job is forbidden to drive, I've been alternating which of our two cars I use. We used his when we went to Chalfont to buy maternity clothes for Carol. She didn't ask me to do it. Buying a maternity outfit for her was something I wanted to do.

Job has been good today, no seizures. But it is obvious that there is some mental deficiency. I had prepared a check for the tax collector and put it and the bill in an envelope and left it on his dresser. We don't mail this bill; we hand carry it to the Township Building. But I put it in the envelope so that he would know it was something I wanted him to look at. I try to keep him abreast of all household transactions. I don't want him to feel shut out of the decision making process. I had also prepared a check for the water and sewer bill. Both items sat together on his dresser. When he thought I was asleep he would pick up first one envelope, then the other, then look at the calendar. He must have repeated those actions at least fifteen times.

He still does things around the house unaided. Today he prepared dinner. Later, he carried crabapples that I had raked up out to the compost pile.

Crickets are chirping into the deepening nighttime. It rained but it has not made the weather any cooler, so the crickets' chirping is loud and lively. It sounds like there are hundreds of them.

SIX

August 22, 1998 (Sunday)

Today was Volunteer Recognition Day at church. Job has been Director of Volunteer Ministries since 1991. He has given up that post and today the church was to honor him. Knowing of his emotional state, I made a special trip to Pastor's office to advise against singling Job out for recognition. I knew he wouldn't want that, I told pastor. "I have known him for over forty years and I have never known him to expect praise for anything he does for his Lord". During the recognition ceremony Pastor did an excellent job of carrying out my wishes. But Pastor Shulz, the former Pastor, had sent Job a beautiful letter through the mail acknowledging gratitude for his faithful, above the call of duty faithfulness.

I had asked Job not to carry the letter with him to the volunteer social, but he did. I was quite annoyed with him. I knew what would happen and had tried to secretly watch to see that he not carry the letter with him. It was private and just to him. He had prepared his own little speech, had spent two days in the preparation of it. And he read it, but then he took from his pocket the letter Pastor had written, and when he started to read it he got all choked up.

Riding along Delmont Avenue I noticed that weeds are starting to turn brown, burned by summer's hot sun. Goldenrod lends color to the browning surrounding. From our bedroom window I watch leaves float down from our crabapple tree. Earlier in the afternoon I tried sitting outside on the patio but it is too sad. Too many memories—of our children playing in the swimming pool, of going to New York to visit Wilma and Steven, of having Job well mentally and physically. Sitting outside makes me sad and I weep. Humidity has returned as a factor in the weather.

I GUESS THAT SUNDAY'S CEREMONY FORMALLY ENDED Job's claim to the title of "Director of Volunteer Ministries". I remember when he assumed the title, 10 years after his heart surgery, and several weeks after his prostate surgery.

He had an epiphany in which he felt God had called him to preach the Gospel. A week after it happened, he told me about it.

"I'm sixty-four-years-old," he said, "I can't go to a seminary at this age, and I don't know what to do."

I did not know what to advise him to do. He was well educated, although not a college graduate. He felt that to work in the Ministry he would need to attend a seminary, and at his age to do so was not practicable. It seemed a shame to me that someone so willing to preach, and who had experienced such a dramatic calling to do so should be denied the opportunity to perform that sacred work because of not having attended a seminary. After all, the only requirement of the Disciples to do the same work was to stop fishing for fish, or stop doing whatever their current work happened to be. Perhaps the Disciples already knew the Greek and Hebrew languages that many seminarians today are required to learn.

Appearing out of sequence, my journal entry for March 18, 1991, provides what may have been the impetus for Job's feeling that he had been called to the Ministry.

March 28, 1991 (Wednesday)

Green grass has completely covered last winter's brown. The wind is up, bending budding trees and evergreens in every direction. Brown leaves that escaped last fall's raking skip across wide lawns and down asphalt-paved streets. How blue the sky is! There are no clouds. When I went out to bring in the paper I felt the warmth from the sun on my face.

Job is still recuperating from the operation to remove the cancer from his prostate. The urologist has given him medicine to stop the "leaking" that is still apparent. I don't trust it not to undo what some of his other medicine controls. I try not to say anything, but I do get concerned.

This operation has been hard on him physically, emotionally, and psychologically. He told me today that last Friday he got so uncontrollably tearful that he felt God had called him to preach. He said he cried and cried, then got on his knees and prayed, and got up and wept some more.

I wonder what message God would have for me if only the tears could flow to express the sadness in my heart: They are always near the surface but seem unable to negotiate the leap over the lump in my throat. Why am I sad? I never know. I think of Job and me, how our lives are so changed from how it used to be.

THAT IS HOW HIS INVOLVEMENT IN VOLUNTEER MINISTRY BEGAN. Since I did not know what advice to offer to help solve his dilemma, I suggested that he talk the matter over with his pastor. He did, and it was Pastor who supplied the idea volunteer ministry as an outlet for his spiritual expression.

Job threw himself wholeheartedly into the work. At first, he would go "up the church" on Mondays and stay for about four hours, working mostly on the computer. Even if we went away for a weekend he felt the need to be back home in time to go to his "ministry" on Monday, devoting more and more time to the work. I began to resent the amount of time that he spent doing what I called "playing with the computer." Data processing was his work. It is what he did to earn a livelihood. He was good at what he did, and he had, I say, single-handedly, convinced the church of not more than two hundred members that they needed a computer.

When I told friends with whom I regularly had lunch about the long hours Job spent at church, they laughingly asked, "What is he doing, putting the whole New Testament on the computer?"

And now, his ministry had ended.

SEVEN

August 24, 1998 (Monday)

I've had a long, busy day. By 5:40 I was up and put in a load of wash. Job came into the kitchen ready for his usual bowl of cereal, but discovered that we had run out of milk. Out of habit, he was readying himself to go to the convenience store to buy some when I reminded him that he wasn't to drive anymore. Oddly, he doesn't seem bothered by lack of that privilege.

Job was to eat lunch before having an EEG test. We ate lunch at the kitchen table, then watched the noon news, which was largely about hurricane Bonnie that is building up but is still out in the ocean. Today has been hot and humid. Newscasters have warned people with respiratory problems to stay indoors.

We went to the hospital and Job had his test. Just as we finished, the neurologist came into the office situated across from the waiting room where we were sitting. Job said he hoped that the test had gone well. The doctor merely replied that he hoped so too. He didn't sound at all encouraging. Maybe I read too much in the tone of his voice, which was rather terse.

Job continues to seem mentally sluggish at home, especially at home. He usually does not initiate conversation, just watches TV but seems not to be following or understanding what is going on. I feel as if my heart will break. Tonight, after darkness came, I sat alone outside and listened to crickets sing.

August 25, 1998 (Tuesday)

I guess this is the time of day that is called dusk. I am sitting outside on the patio. It is cool outside, but inside it is a bit sticky. Job and I watched the Jim Lehrer News Hour together. He did not come outside with me.

In the late afternoon clouds gathered and a few drops of rain fell as I sat at the table that is in the circle where the above ground pool used to be. There is no threat of rain now. Where the sun is setting, a spot of clear blue sky separates dark blue clouds from dark gray ones. Down the street in this always quiet, suburban neighborhood, a dog is barking. I don't think it's Donnie's dog, I'm not familiar with this dog's bark. The thunderous roar of a military airplane from the Naval Air Base just rose to a great crescendo and is now dying away in the distance. All of our beds of phlox are dying. Marigolds are starting to bloom.

August 26, 1998 (Wednesday)

It would seem that I would have lots of time to rest, but there is always something to be done. Job is not getting any better. Sometimes he seems just fine, but he is very stubborn. He won't do anything that I suggest for him to try in order to stimulate his brain. Tonight, he went to church to help get the newsletter together. It is a project that he used to coordinate. I drove him to church. Jane Adams brought him home for me. He never talks to me except to ask a question about something. I am afraid it is Alzheimer's and that the time will come when I cannot care for him. It has been very hot today. In the evening I put the air conditioner on so that the bedroom would be comfortable.

August 28, 1998 (Friday)

Today has been better for us. Job seems more upbeat and has actually talked to me. He hasn't even asked too many questions, the same ones, over, and over again. I was up early, anxious to get on with my jelly making. I waited, though, until Job finished his breakfast. I didn't want to rush him. I saw our neighbor walking by the ditch and suggested that Job go over and chat with him. He did. We went out to lunch. On the way, we dropped off Job's prescription for his "memory pills." I asked the druggist what he thought of the medicine, and he said, "It works."

When we got home I read the fact sheet that describes what the medicine is for and what the side effects of taking it are. The fact sheet disclosed that the medicine, Aricept, is used to treat Alzheimer's disease. So, I guess that is what Job has.

August 29, 1998 (Saturday)

Move along August, out to eternity, or wherever months go when the year doesn't need them anymore. Today is fitness center day. While there Job had a mild state of confusion. He couldn't remember whether he had worked out on the UBE, and was unwilling to go on to another piece of equipment. He finally did move on.

Maybe the memory pills are working. Job has no memory of the day that he got so confused that he had to go to our doctor and from there to the emergency room of the hospital. Yet, this evening, hours after the occasion of the incident, he remembered how confused he got this morning.

He kept talking about it, so I said to him, "At least you remember that it happened. That's progress."

We went to rent a video. I guess the plethora of visual stimuli surrounding him in the store was too much of an assault on his brain. He became so confused trying to help me make a selection he couldn't speak. I realized immediately what was wrong and quickly hustled him out of the store, where he sat in the car and waited for me. I feel so alone, and I am so tired.

September 1, 1998 (Tuesday)

There is no trace of August left. September came right in favoring September. August helped, for the weather turned cool before midnight. Today is a cool September day, presaging fall. Clear, blue sky abounds. Broken down, white, fluffy clouds roam the sky. After fitness center I was inside all morning typing Marty's nursery school class list. Wilma has been dead since July, but I can't get her image from my mind.

Job has been good all day, until this afternoon. Since I had been busy all day, I left dinner for him to prepare. Notes were available on how to do every item of preparation. I was in the bedroom when I heard him complaining agitatedly to himself. I went to the kitchen to investigate. He couldn't get the tomato peeled. I told him that I would do it. I did, and finished preparing the rest of dinner, cleaned up the kitchen, and we sat down and ate. There was a time when he would have berated me for not first pouring hot water over the tomato to make peeling it easier.

September 2, 1998 (Wednesday)

Today has been a bad day for Job, in the morning at least. We were to go to the supermarket, and he, as he always has done, was making out his shopping list. We only needed to buy a few items, milk and the like. I was at the word processor typing. Job grew quiet and stopped asking me questions. I sensed trouble and went into the bedroom, where I found him crying. When I asked what was the matter, he said he was confused. I tried to determine the source of his confusion but was unable to. He said he felt help-less. I told him to go into the bathroom and wash his face. He finally did, but first he lay on the bathroom floor crying.

It was very distressing for me. I wanted to call someone, our children, maybe, the doctor, but what would I say to him, or them? Finally, I called no one, deciding that it was my cross to bear.

Clouds had hung about all day and I suggested that the gloomy weather might be the cause of his depression. He finally got himself together and we went to the supermarket. He was okay for the rest of the day, but when in the afternoon I asked him how he felt, he said, "Okay, but I still have a feeling of anx-iety."

Worrying about Job, and thinking about Wilma, gives rise to a lump in my throat. If only there were a place where I could go and scream and no one would hear.

In the evening I carried Marty's typed material to her. We talked about Job. She said I could always call her or Bob if I need to talk to someone.

September 3, 1998 (Thursday)

After last night's rain, today has been deliciously cool. Most of the day I spent going to the hairdresser, getting my hair done, and driving home again. Job has seemed okay today, except he didn't take the T-shirt that he exercised in off. The sleeves of it protruded from under the short-sleeved shirt that he put on over it. That is not his usual way of dressing, but today he seemed comfortable with it.

September 4, 1998 (Friday)

With morning chores done, we went to Old Mill Inn for

lunch, I had intended to stop by the bank after we left the restaurant, but Job didn't feel well. We went to Chalfont and exchanged Carol's maternity dress. I'll take the new one to her when we go out to Ohio next week. The weather has been beautiful, only a little sticky.

Tiredness descended upon me like a whirlwind once nightfall came. I went to bed early. Job was still up and I could hear him doing something until after 11:00. He put the TV on but didn't stay in the room to watch the program.

September 5, 1998 (Saturday)

Move along September, toward Labor Day, toward end of summer, toward my seventieth birthday, toward the end of the year. I wouldn't have gone to the fitness center, but Job wanted to go, and he can't drive anymore. Afterwards, I went alone to Perkins for breakfast. When I came home I lay down and napped, wasting a beautiful, beautiful day. When I awoke I heard Job and our neighbor talking on our patio. They visited for a long time. I hope Job's responses to conversation were appropriate.

September 7, 1998 (Labor Day)

The day broke clear and beautiful; the temperature went to 90 degrees. We had no plans for doing anything. No one would visit us. We would visit no one. I did regular household things. I have a feeling of heaviness in my chest. Am I about to have a flare-up of sarcoidosis? I certainly hope not. The Prednisone that I must take to combat it makes me so fat. Tonight I threw out the pills that were prescribed for me in 1995 and that I continued to take until sometime in 1996 when I was weaned off having to take them.

September 9, 1998 (Wednesday)

This September day is clear, and cool. The wind is blowing gently, unhinging leaves from their summer home. It is early morning, not yet 9:30, but Job has already brought my breakfast. I sat in the bedroom and ate. I feel better today but am despondent. I look out of our window and think of things that happened long, long ago. I'm short-winded. We should go food shopping today, but maybe we won't. Job went out to the vegetable garden and when he came in he was all out of breath.

September 10, 1998 (Thursday)
Last night it turned quite chilly, making it difficult to get out of bed and to the fitness center by 6:00. I did a shorter time on each piece of equipment. Even so, by midday I am tired and usually take a long, hard-to-wake-up-from nap. I still have a dry cough that troubles me. Things seem to be going well for Job. He is keeping on top of things and hasn't had a crying jag for the past week. Things seem almost normal. The nation is focused on the Special Counsel's report on President Clinton.

September 11, 1998 (Friday)
It was quite chilly when we got up. It is a little warmer now. The day is clear and beautiful. Fall is not here yet, although today's weather makes it seem like fall. Job worked outside for a while, mowing the lawn and cleaning up the compost pile. I thoroughly cleaned the rec. room. We've watched the noon news. I think we'll ride down to the mall just for a change of pace.

September 13, 1998 (Sunday)
Sundays are long. There's nothing to do. We went to church. The preacher preached. I have no idea about what. For most of the day Job and I were in separate places. He sat outside reading the newspaper. I was in our bedroom. At night, Amy called. I'm glad. I had wanted to call her and Carol but decided against it. I don't like to intrude myself into their lives too frequently.

September 14, 1998 (Monday)
Today is another hot day. I kept busy, too busy. I should relax more. Job puttered in the yard. I'm glad to see him do that.

September 16, 1998 (Wednesday)
We left at 10:50 to go to Cincinnati to visit Carol and Aaron. We are going to spend a week with them. Carol did a lot to make our stay enjoyable, even though she didn't feel well many days because of her pregnancy.

September 23, 1998 (Wednesday)

We're home now. Today is a perfect first day of fall. It is chilly. Brisk is a better description of the weather. It is sunny, making the sky bright and blue. Job mowed the lawn. Everything has the look of fall. Tomorrow is Job's big day. We go to the neurologist for the results of his EEG that was taken in August.

EIGHT

September 24, 1998 (Thursday)

This is our big day. We've waited a month for it to come. How will we feel? What will we do when the verdict is in?

We overslept a little and didn't get up until 6:00 to head for the fitness center. We were anxious to get there and home again and eat breakfast. Our appointment with the neurologist, Dr. Howard, was for 10:30. We arrived about 10 minutes early and were allowed to go right in to see the doctor. He shook our hand. We sat in his office and he told us the result of the EEG that Job had taken in August. That seems so long ago, so far away from present.

The EEG test determined that since Job had not suffered a series of mini strokes to cause his forgetfulness, the diagnosis is that he has Alzheimer's disease. We took the news calmly. What else could we do? His medication, Aricept, was increased from 5mgs to 10mgs. When we carried the prescription to the pharmacist he told us that the dosage was the highest that can ever be prescribed.

We had an appointment to attend a seminar that was in a building close by the doctor's office. The seminar was on the importance of wills. We must get ours updated. How long will it be before Job's mind deteriorates totally? He is okay now. What else can happen to him? This afternoon he raked up crabapples. He keeps busy.

THREE YEARS HAVE PASSED since that last journal entry. Thinking back, I do not remember if the doctor told us about the different stages of the disease. I can only remember that at his suggestion we made an appointment to see him in six months, a pattern that until recently we have followed. Very recently it has become necessary to see him more often. In the meantime, over the most recent years, I have come to know in a very painful way just what else can happen, and indeed has happened to my beloved.

September 25, 1998 (Friday)
It is cloudy today. I did some early morning chores and got them out of the way by noontime. Job cleaned up the breakfast dishes. When he knew I was finished the housework, he said he would like to go to a mall. I knew why. Sunday is my birthday. We went to the mall in Willow Grove. I was afraid to let him out of my sight. I also encouraged him to not look too intensely for a gift for me. I was afraid too much mental exertion would cause him to become confused. With my help, he bought a belt that I really wanted. We had lunch in the food court. I ate a hot-dog. He drank a fruit punch.

While we were eating he remembered that he had bought a birthday card for me while we were in Cincinnati. I was so proud of him for making that far away recall. I am also glad that he thought to get one while he and Carol were together. I remember now that I sat in the car while the two of them went into the card store. He's cooking dinner now. I'm watching the news.

September 27, 1998 (Sunday)
Today I reached the age of the biblical threescore and ten. I feel tired, but no more tired or older than I did yesterday. I got up early so that I could take Job to Sunday school. I knew he would want to go. I stayed myself, although I probably will not go back. There is not much time spent discussing things interactively. The new pastor loves to talk. Also, nothing was discussed that helped me with my dilemma of how to increase my faith so that I am assured of a hereafter in heaven. At seventy, I feel that I should KNOW that my house is in order.

It has been very hot today. In some places the temperature went to 90 degrees and beyond, breaking, or equaling a record set for the date in 1881.

The card Job gave me is beautiful. Amy also sent a nice one. Lois called, so did Carol. Carol is feeling better. I'm glad. It is night. The neighborhood, except for the quiet song of a few crickets, is absolutely silent.

September 28, 1998 (Monday)

What a beautiful day it is. The brightness of sunshine, the blueness of sky, and the briskness of blowing wind abstracts from this end-of-September-day its true character and gives it the look of one borrowed from October.

I was up first, before 6:00, I think. I brought the paper in, and while drinking my orange juice and coffee, did the cryptogram and jumble puzzles. I sat down to relax and while doing so went through a box of clippings that I've kept on a shelf in my closet for years. The clippings were of nothing important, just report cards from the girls' school years, a few receipts, and other tidbits. Together they tell a story of sorts. I tied the box back up and put it back on the shelf.

Job did piddling things in the yard. Time was he would have gone "up to the church." I think there are things he could still do, but because the former Pastor is not there he has no desire to do them.

September 29, 1998 (Tuesday)

Job and I went to the bank where our safe deposit box is located and brought home the contents of the box. We must get things squared away, update our wills, and make appropriate designations of our assets. It is so much trouble, and Job is absolutely no help. It has been another beautiful day, but I was so busy I didn't get outside much to enjoy it. I am always busy.

September 30, 1998 (Wednesday)

Goodbye, September. You served me well. You brought me to another year and started me on the way to still another one. Your weather has been spectacular. You also brought some relief for President Clinton. The last few weeks have shown the public and Democratic Congressmen giving him more support.

Today I went to the hairdresser. I felt badly leaving Job alone for so long. Before I left to come home I called to see if he was okay. After I got home we went to the food market. He cooked dinner. Lois called to tell me that one of her friends has died. His wife has Alzheimer's and is in a nursing home. I hope Job never has to go into a home. I am going to care for him as long as I can. Right now he's okay, but how long will it be before he isn't? No one knows. He didn't tolerate the higher dosage of Aricept. Does that mean that his brain will deteriorate in a shorter time?

Last night I had a good, solid dream about Wilma. She was her fat, healthy-looking self. And whatever was going on wherever she is, she was happy. I could tell because she had a big smile on her face, the kind I saw so many times.

NINE

❦

ERIODIC BREAKS IN CHRONOLOGICAL JOURNAL ENTRIES indicate
that nothing significant relating to Job's Alzheimer's disease
was recorded. If mention is made of him, it is in connection with his doing ordinary things that he would have done had
he not been afflicted with the disease.

October 21, 1998 (Wednesday)
On Monday Job had appointments with our primary care
physician, Dr Miles, and with his urologist. Today we went to his
cardiologist. That's it for doctor visits until our dental appointments in December. I am so very lonely. Job is hardly any company at all. Sometimes his responses to my attempt to make conversation are contentious. I try to help him by suggesting things to do
that might stimulate his memory, but it is very, very difficult.

October 31, 1998 (Halloween)
Oh, October, must you go, carrying with you your clear, blue
skies and colorful foliage? Past days have been warm and beautiful.
Leaves fall in flurries. The ones on the silver maple directly
behind the house have all almost fallen off. The ones on the
maple between Palladino, our neighbor, and us are yellowing and
beginning to fall. But the ones on the maple between our other
neighbor and us are still green and hanging on tenaciously.
I had planned to go to a mall and spend some money to help
the sagging economy, but at the fitness center Job had one of his
incidents, a hard one.
I had just finished my time on the treadmill and was beginning to do the rower when by chance I looked back. Job was on

the treadmill directly behind me. It must have been a sixth sense that made me look back. I saw that he was in distress and rushed to him. The technician in charge of the floor also came over and made a chair available for Job, and he sat and rested. Afterwards we came home. Neither of us did any more of our workout.

Job ate his usual "king's" breakfast but fell asleep while sitting at the table reading the newspaper. Eventually, he decided to get into bed. He slept for a long time. When he finally got up he said he felt fine, but he remembered almost nothing of what transpired earlier.

November 11, 1998 (Veterans' Day)
Our cousin in South Carolina died, and my brother Angelo and I would have driven down for the funeral, but we had just been to the doctor and Job's blood pressure was elevated, so the doctor advised against making the trip.

I don't know what is wrong with Job. He is quiet, and often irritable.

THE ARGUMENT COULD BE MADE, I suppose, that since I knew that Job's condition was Alzheimer's, I should have known to expect the behaviors that he was presenting. But I did not know what to expect, because, except for one overall warning about the condition, I had not been alerted to expect the personality transformation in Job that I was witnessing.

The neurologist did tell us that at some point Job's mind could deteriorate to where he would not be able to speak or perform any of the actions that depend on the brain for direction.

In time, at least two years from the time these behaviors were occurring, I would come to know that mood swings, losing things, depression, and others peculiarities are characteristic of the disease. But if our doctors forewarned us that these drastic changes in behavior would occur, I do not remember hearing them. I am very positive that I had no written information on the subject of Alzheimer's disease.

What I remember vividly, and it might have been as early in the disease as these journal entries, is that our hammer disappeared from Job's workbench. I searched and searched every place I felt a hammer could hang or lay, but at least a year passed before

I stumbled upon it in a most (I don't remember where) unlikely place. The drain to the kitchen sink disappeared and to this day has not been found. Needless to say, a new one was bought to replace it, and I watch whenever Job heads for the compost pile in case he has it with him. I have a strong suspicion that that was the fate of the lost one.

November 15, 1998 (Sunday)
How wonderful it is to have another lovely, warm day. Everywhere I drive there is beautiful fall foliage. I wore only a lightweight jacket over my dress to church. After church Job and I had a big row about his medications. I had given him the opportunity to be responsible for taking them, explaining that that was one thing I wanted him to do for as long as possible. The problem is, he does not believe me when I tell him which medicine is which, and he takes at least five different ones. It was a big row. I called Lois and told her that I'm sure he'll have a sick spell tomorrow.

November 16, 1998 (Monday)
As I predicted, he did have an "incident". We had been to the optician to get a screw put back in his eyeglasses. On our way home we stopped to pick up the prescription we had left at the druggist's on Friday and did a few other errands. Neither of us had had much to say to each other today, a result of yesterday's row.

We sat in our bedroom as we usually do. He had the newspaper to read. I was going to read a book. Almost immediately, I heard Job gasping for breath and holding his head. I asked him if he was all right, or did he want to lie down. He said he wasn't sure if he should lie down or continue sitting in his recliner. He ended up sitting in the chair and sleeping for about an hour. By the time I was ready to leave to go to dinner with friends, he seemed okay.

It would be a long time before I would come to realize that his sudden attacks of some seeming distress were his way of getting the positive rather than negative attention that he wanted.

November 17, 1998 (Tuesday)
I was awake early; Job was not. I let him sleep. It was half

past six when he awoke. At the fitness center, I was pleased that Job's blood pressure was one hundred forty over something reasonable. We completed our equipment without incident. Job doesn't do the treadmill anymore.

It has been a good day. It is cloudy, but not a dreary cloudy. You can tell that the sun is lurking close to the surface. Job cleaned the front and back gutters of accumulated leaves. Now it is 9:15 and he has been incident free. Oops, just this minute I saw him slinking down. I asked him what the trouble was and he said he felt weak and his stomach felt funny. He's done a lot of eructating. I'd say it was something he had for dinner, except the same thing happened yesterday and he hadn't eaten anything. It's 9:30 now. His sick spell seems to be over. He is in bed reading. I hate being alone with him when it is night and he is sick. I never know what to do. I cannot call the doctor every time he has a sick spell, although when I've mentioned the occurrence of them to the doctor he examines him and can find nothing physical that causes them.

November 18 1998 (Wednesday)
Job had another "attack" today. He was preparing his breakfast when it happened. He sat at the table for a few moments but decided to get back into bed. He didn't undress. He slept for a couple of hours. I prepared his breakfast, and later, lunch, and still later, dinner. He has been in our bedroom for most of the day. I joined him there for dinner. All day I have been busy caring for him. I had planned to go to Wrightstown and work on Amy's quilt, but there was no time for that. I raked the last big dropping of leaves from our maple trees. Now there will be just raking the gleanings and the yard will be clear for winter.

I wonder if I am losing Job. I feel very alone.

November 28, 1998 (Saturday)
Spent Thanksgiving with Amy and James. We went to James' parents for Thanksgiving dinner. Ummm. What delicious food, and plenty of it.

December 2, 1998 (Wednesday)
The temperature went to 61 degrees today. I carried Job to get

a prescription filled. At home, I sat at the picnic table and ate lunch. I saw a dandelion in bloom as if it were its season for being. A few yellow jackets and flies still fly lazily about. Blue sky is garnished with wisps of silky, elongated, white clouds. The grass is still springtime green, but trees are bare. November knew its job and did it.

Last night and tonight I practiced the piano. I never get anything to tempo, but I am pleased that I can read and execute the notes.

December 13, 1998 (Sunday)

The House Judiciary Committee has been debating whether to impeach President Clinton. I've been caught up in it emotionally, and both Job and I have spent a lot of time in the rec. room watching the proceedings.

While not in the 70's, the weather is quite warm. I try to think of what we did at this time of the year when the children were at home, and of the years when they were away at school. I can't remember. Time, once it is gone, is gone forever. It looks like Christmas is coming, but it doesn't feel that way.

On Friday we bought a live tree, a little one, that can be placed on a table. Job trimmed it. I think he was glad to do that. I remember when he reluctantly gave the trimming of the tree over to the children. I never had much interest in tree trimming, although I've enjoyed putting other decorations up.

This year I've not done much of that. A centerpiece comprised of candles adorns the dining room table. I have bought one poinsettia, which is on the accent table in front of the bow window.

December 23, 1998 (Wednesday)

The day has gotten off to a bad start. I went out and brought the newspaper in and was sitting at the kitchen table reading and having my coffee when Job came in dressed for going to the fitness center. He asked me if I was going, and I replied that tomorrow was our day to go, and we would go then. He went into the bathroom and started a crying spell that carried over into our bedroom. I decided to ignore him and went on with my work. Eventually he came out to the kitchen and prepared his breakfast. For the rest of the day he was fine. We went to the supermarket,

I made pies for Christmas dinner; he put in the remaining storm windows.

The house is decorated, not like other years, but it does look nice. Other houses in our block, and around the neighborhood have lights on outside. We used to have them as well, but this year when he tried to get the lights up, Job got very confused, so our house is bare of outside decorations.

I haven't heard much Christmas music on the radio. Tonight we've watched the Mormon Tabernacle Choir singing Christmas music. We've also listened to and watched the Atlanta Symphony Orchestra on television. Two separate choral groups, conducted by Robert Shaw, sang.

December 24, 1998 (Christmas Eve)

Christmas Eve already! Once it started to come, it came quickly. I've had a full day. I had to go to the city to pick Lois up. Amy and James arrived. I cooked dinner. Amy and James went to visit Amy's friend, Jill. Surprisingly, Job did not want to go to church service. I am going to put my gifts under the tree and go to bed.

December 25, 1998 (Christmas Day)

Job was Elder for today's church service. I drove him to church but didn't stay for the service. When he came home we all ate breakfast together. Later there was dinner and conversation. Lois, James, Job, and I played the game "Clue." James won. Because of her pregnancy (she's due in February), I had advised Carol not to come home for the holiday, even though I knew that she wanted to be with us. Carol's absence and Wilma's passing earlier in the year made this Christmas very sad for all of us. Everyone made an effort to conceal his true feelings, but the lie of the effort's success was glaring.

December 29, 1998 (Tuesday)

Fast away the Old Year passes. It has been dreary all day. Sometimes, it rained, a steady drizzly rain. We went for our workout at the fitness center. I spent most of the afternoon writing thank-you notes for gifts that the nursery school children had given me for Christmas. I sat down in the recliner to take a nap.

When I awoke Job was preparing dinner. We're still eating Christmas turkey. Maybe tomorrow I will get it stored in the freezer. I wish Job were not slipping away from me. This year has been bad enough, and what will 1999 bring?

December 31, 1998 (Thursday)

While Job ate breakfast after we came from the fitness center, I began dismantling the Christmas tree. I didn't get the ornaments put away; maybe I will get that done tomorrow. I did get the refrigerator cleared of left over turkey and threw out little bits of foods that will not be eaten. It has been a typical end-of-the-year-day. A little sunshine shone through winter gray clouds that at times let through some blue sky.

As always, I hate to see the ending of the Old Year. This year we discovered that Job has Alzheimer's, Carol became pregnant, and Amy got married.

TEN

A S THE NEW YEAR BEGINS, it will not only mean turning the pages on another year of life, it will mean turning the pages of the journal on which I have recorded the mundane as well as some relevant occurrences in my life. What is written is not in formal journals, but in ordinary five-subject composition books. And, just as what each day will bring to our lives is held a mystery until it happens, so are the contents of each journal entry unknown until I turn the page to a new date.

The journals were begun over thirty-five years ago, when I needed to write down the feelings I was experiencing when I knew that a new life, that of our second daughter, was being formed within my body. I felt the need to record everything about those moments. As years go by, I forget what was written at a given time until the entry is re-read. I know that the entries for 1999 will contain things about Job's mental deterioration, but I will not remember the behavioral changes that occurred until they are recalled by reading my journal notes.

January 1, 1999 (Friday)

What a beautiful beginning of the year today is. It is cold. The sky is blue with fluffy, white clouds scattered about. Our neighborhood, as always, is quiet. Job has been quiet, quiet, quiet all day. I've just left him alone. I did get him to accompany me to the store. I needed leeks for the lentil soup that I decided to make, and I didn't have any.

January 5, 1999 (Tuesday)

I thought Job would be sick today, because last night we had a row about hooking up our new answering machine. Sometimes I have to fight back to preserve my own sanity. He's okay, though, and we've been busy doing little things. He cooked a delicious dinner. The difficulty arises when he does not realize his limitations. For instance, even before he tried to install the new machine, I knew that he wouldn't be able to do it. I also knew that he would try and might possibly get something out of order that I would not know how to make right again.

January 7, 1999 (Thursday)

Snow had been predicted for last night. We lay snugly in bed dreading to relinquish that comfort for dressing to go to the fitness center. Finally, I asked Job to go and look out of the window to see what the conditions for driving were. I don't drive if there is any possibility of ice.

Before Christmas, we would look at the digital clock radio on Job's nightstand to check the time. But that one was thrown out (I kept it, however) by Job in favor of the little electric clock that Brian Adams had given him as a gift. Brian had hosted the elders and their wives at a Christmas social. His wife Jane had given the ladies a recipe book, and Brian had given each elder a small, electric clock.

Job has had difficulty telling the time with the new clock. Was it a quarter of five or a quarter of six, he asked? While he was looking out of the window, I told him the time, and he began to try to say something about it: "It's a quarter to 6, quarter to fff, si—", and I heard a thud.

He had fallen to the floor. I jumped out of bed and rushed to help him up. I don't know what caused him to fall. There was nothing in the way to cause him to trip. If he became unconscious, he recovered in seconds. He went to the front door and opened it. It was very cold, and he only had on pajamas. I was afraid he had gone outside, but by the time I got to the front of the house he had already started back toward the bedroom. I noticed that he was staggering and was sure that he had suffered a stroke.

I insisted that he go back to bed. We debated whether to call the doctor and decided against doing so. That was a good decision, I guess, because for the rest of the day he was fine, almost.

Sometime later he got out of bed and began looking for the brush that cleans his razor head.

I was practically sure that the brush was in his travel kit and told him to look there for it, but he refused to do so. He searched, and searched, over and over again in the most unlikely places. Finally he stopped searching. When I had time, I looked in the travel case, got out the brush, and put it in the medicine cabinet where he keeps his razor.

January 8, 1999 (Friday)

It is overcast. I think it will snow. Job is in a crying mood today. I heard him in the bathroom weeping and went to see if there was anything I could do. He said there was not, that he was just confused. The confusion, I think, stemmed from the fact that the razor brush was where he could see it. I didn't say anything. He cried and cried for a long time, and I let him. I have learned that there is nothing that I can do. Eventually he came out to the kitchen and prepared his breakfast.

I had set everything out for him in an effort to relieve him of any confusion. Without anyone advising me, I have concluded that the cause for some of his confusion is the mental exertion of trying to fit things into some proper order.

[Down the road from the present time, I will discover that my reasoning is to some degree correct.

For instance, to prepare his breakfast he must think about getting the cereal down from the shelf, and think about where in the kitchen the cereal is located. Likewise, he must think about what is needed to go with the cereal. Ah, milk. Then, he must think about where the milk is located, and so on with every item he must use in preparing his meal.

The individual not suffering from Alzheimer's disease (or other dementia) performs automatically the steps necessary to accomplish a simple task like preparing one's breakfast.]

In the afternoon we played a game of Scrabble. He won, and I was actually pleased about it. In past years, I would not have been pleased with his success. He was very good at the game, beating me sometimes when I held several bonus tiles.

Snow did come. I shoveled out our driveway. Donnie came over with his father's snow blower and helped.

January 10, 1999 (Saturday)

The snow will probably be around for a while, even though we had rain today. This afternoon a gusty wind has blown. Our streets and driveways are clear. This morning there was some ice around the car but driving wasn't bad. Job's blood pressure was a little high at the beginning and end of exercising. Michael had him do an extra cool-down lap, and it was better. Tonight just after dinner, he was sick. This is the second time this week. It is so worrisome.

January 11, 1999 (Monday)

We are sending the crib that both Carol and Amy used as babies to Carol. That's exciting. Job had to climb up into the attic to get it. I was concerned about him climbing around up there, but he was okay. We carried it to UPS to have it shipped to Cincinnati. When we got home there was a call on the machine from Dr. Miles saying we could pick up the letter to PenDot letting them know that Job isn't to drive anymore. By the time that was done, it was time to start dinner.

January 12, 1999 (Tuesday)

Something is wrong with Job, but I don't know what. Other than Alzheimer's, apparently the doctors don't either. At the fitness center, I saw him sitting instead of using the equipment. I asked the technician to check on him for me. Michael did and said Job's blood pressure had dropped and he felt faint. We didn't do any more workout, just came home, and I prepared his breakfast. I no longer get upset. I just wait for whatever is going to happen to happen. Our only outing on this beautiful day has been to the drugstore to pick up his prescription.

January 13, 1999 (Wednesday)

This has not been a good day for Job. When he was getting washed, he thinks he got as far as brushing his teeth when he discovered that his stomach was in knots. I brought a basin of water and helped him finish his bath. He has stayed in our bedroom all day. I brought his meals there.

IN RETROSPECT, I BELIEVE THESE SPELLS OF SICKNESS for which the doctors could find no physical cause were anxiety attacks. They never told me that, but in writings that I have come into possession of as the disease has progressed I learned that anxiety is a factor in Alzheimer's sufferers.

January 17, 1999 (Sunday)
It is another day of sunshine and melting snow. We went to Grace church. Job stayed for Assembly meeting, but I came home. I wanted to go to the city to visit Lois but knew it would be too late when Job came home from church. I walked out to the back of our yard. Snow crunched under my feet as I walked. I was out for a long time, just walking around. A flock of geese flew overhead. A lump came to my throat.

January 21, 1999 (Thursday)
We got a late start going to market. After the food was put away we went to the rec. room to watch President Clinton's lawyers present their case against his impeachment.
It has been overcast today. These types of days seem especially hard for Job. He doesn't seem to remember anything for more than a second.

January 27, 1999 (Wednesday)
I feel sluggish today as I try to fight off the second day of sinus discomfort. Job's sister Gwen called him today. She hardly ever calls him. During the course of their conversation I heard him ask about her husband Stanford who has been dead for about six years. Job is just okay. His eyes, once so lively and bright, look sick. The whites look dull, and the sparkle has gone out of the brown.

February 9, 1999 (Tuesday)
For Christmas I gave Job two calendars that allow each day to be torn away. To me, the calendars are quickly getting thinner. Tearing pages from those calendars each day makes it seem like the year is passing away more rapidly than usual. I bought the calendars hoping they would help him keep track of the days. It is not working. He doesn't look at the calendars. I am the one who rips the spent day's date away.

He was sick for a while on Sunday and again yesterday. He seems okay—today. It was the same malady—funny feeling in his head and a distressful stomach. Last night as we lay in bed I heard him crying. When I asked why, he said he felt confused. He said sometimes he goes into the kitchen and doesn't even know where to find a glass. I think I am beyond getting upset about it. I live with it. Today he seems fine.

February 16, 1999 (Tuesday)

It is evening. This is the second day of my intermittent, two-day sinus attack. I was awake by 4:00 AM, at times very ill. I sat at the kitchen table with my head bowed. Job was up by 6:00 and wanted to know if I felt up to going to the fitness center. I didn't, but we did go. We were home by 9:00.

It has been a beautiful day, quite warm. Daffodils are shooting up. The temperature went to 60 degrees, I think. Our only outing was a trip to the bank, the drugstore, and the post office. It was a nice outing. In the morning I had done lots of ironing. It was noon before I finished and was able to go out.

Dinner was ready by 5:00. I do the cooking now. Job doesn't offer anymore. Once a few weeks ago he said he would get dinner together, but when I came up from the rec. room he had done nothing except make a pot of tea. He said he was confused.

A while ago this evening I sat in the living room on the couch. I rarely sit in there. It is quiet and lonely. There are no signs, and only vague memories of times when the room was full of life with children playing and my sisters telephoning. Now, it is quiet. This morning I heard birds singing. I wish my headache would go away. I need to feel well. I called Carol. The doctor has told her that progress toward readiness for the baby's delivery is proceeding slowly.

February 18, 1999 (Thursday)

Today we became grandparents. I had gone to the nursery school. When I got home at 2:00, Job was talking on the telephone to his sister Gwen telling her that Carol had given birth to a baby boy. Once he was off the phone, I called Carol right away. Aaron answered, but I talked to Carol. The baby was delivered by Caesarean section and weighed 6 pounds and I forget the ounces. I'm concerned that he must spend the night in Children's hospital because of something that happened during the delivery. But Carol has been given assurance by doctors that little Julian Alexander Durr is going to be all right.

February 22, 1999 (Monday)

Today would be my father's birthday. He passed away long ago, but I always remember his birthday. We've been calling Cincinnati a lot. At first I thought the baby was only mildly sick, but I know now that he could be in serious trouble. Carol went home yesterday. The baby is still in the hospital. When she called today she said he is off all medications, tubes have been removed, he is alert, and is learning how to eat. Tomorrow we fly out to see him.

ELEVEN

March 16, 1999 (Tuesday)

We've been visiting Carol. When we arrived in Cincinnati little Julian was still in the hospital. His doctor had promised that he could come home the next day. When they decided to keep him another day, Carol cried and said she wanted him home with her. I told her that she didn't want to bring him home until he was really well and tried to reassure her that he would be fine.

March 18, 1999 (Thursday)

Job prepared most of the dinner today. He hasn't done that since sometime in January.

March 19, 1999 (Friday)

Today has been a good day. It is frightening. Job came out to the kitchen dressed for church. I didn't call attention to his error. Eventually he realized it himself. He didn't get upset, just laughed about it and changed his clothes. He helped me with the cleaning. While I cleaned the bathrooms, he vacuumed. For the second day in a row, he prepared dinner. As I said, it's frightening.

March 23, 1999 (Tuesday)

Yesterday we went to the neurologist. He wasn't very encouraging about Job's condition. He's rather non-committal anyway. He informed us that since our last visit in September, Job has lost some cognitive capability. The doctor determines this by the tests that are administered during our office visit. He wasn't too impressed when I informed him that I tried reducing Job's confusion by making things available for him so that the stress of searching for them is eliminated.

March 27, 1999 (Saturday)
    Job had a very bad day today. I still am not feeling well because of a cold, so we didn't go to the fitness center. I don't know if that is what set him off or not. I went into the kitchen for my usual cup of coffee. I heard him crying and mumbling to himself while in the bathroom. All day he has been confused about one thing or another and has been generally disagreeable.

March 28, 1999 (Palm Sunday)
    Job seems much better today. He probably doesn't remember yesterday at all. We went to church today. I prepared a nice dinner. Keeping up a tradition we started when the children were home, we always eat Sunday dinner in the dining room rather than the kitchen.
    Job doesn't talk much. He sits with the TV Guide in hand and often looks at the clock to see what the next program is. It has been cold today, and cloudy. Yesterday I talked to Carol. I feel so alone, so ready to weep.

April 6, 1999 (Tuesday)
    Things have been going well with Job lately. His blood pressure is stable, and mentally, he is holding his own. Today we walked to the back of our yard where the apple trees are and marveled at the number of flowers that are on them. Job said he would spray the trees so that the fruit won't be blighted.

CHANGES IN JOB'S CONDITION continue to be gradual. Large skips in journal entries indicate that nothing different is happening in his behavior, and whatever journal entries I've made during those unrecorded days are more my daily musings than a chronicle of his cognitive decline.
    I know that there are stages of the disease, the least distressing being "early cognitive decline". I presume, but am not sure, that he is still in the early stage. Like an ostrich, I bury my head in the sand and refuse to inquire of the neurologist whether he has progressed beyond that point.
    Now, in fact, is a good time to get to know him as he was, not

handsome, but good looking, clean cut, and neat. His build was slight, but his clothes fit well. I would learn later that he had a brilliant mind. He was a gentleman, gentle, and loving. These things you should know before the beast that has hold of him drags him to another stage of dementia, and before I start to forget that he ever possessed those and many other wonderful attributes.

TWELVE

Where do I begin,
To tell the story of how great a love can be
The sweet love story that is older than the sea
The simple truth about the love she (he) brings to me?
Where do I start?

THE BEGINNING GOES BACK ALMOST FIFTY YEARS, but we've been married for only forty-five, had been married for forty-two when the dementia began. I saw his name years before I saw his face. In our church, the African Methodist Episcopal, we had yearly Sunday school conventions. Today, what was known as Sunday schools back then are called church schools now, I believe. The conventions were a gathering of young people who were interested in learning more about the religious beliefs of their church in a setting other than regular morning worship service.

The cluster of churches in our District would send one or more delegates to the convention. His membership was in one church, mine in another. I was very involved in my Sunday school, and was chosen to be a delegate to the convention from my early teens and into my twenties. He was a delegate also, but we never seemed to be at the same session of the Convention at the same time.

Then, a time came when not only were we both delegates, we both were scheduled to participate in a panel discussion titled, "How to Choose a Life Mate."

That was the beginning of what was to become a very special relationship. I observed that he was relaxed and confident when involved in discussions within a group, but on a one-on-

one basis he was very shy.

I saw him at various Youth Group functions from time to time during the year after we met at the Convention. But a full year would pass from the time of our first meeting until he asked me out on a date. We went on a triple date with his two older brothers. One brother was already married and was accompanied by his wife. The brother closest to him in age was with his date. We went to an amusement park. I enjoyed being with him on this Fourth of July holiday.

Subsequent dates were less far apart and were frequent enough that in the vernacular of the day we could be said to be "going steady". Our personalities were similar in so many ways that we were very comfortable together. Where he was shy, I was more so, although people generally regarded my shyness as being aloof. I could hardly have been more inaccurately characterized.

I cannot account for why I was ill at ease with people, even family members, I only know that being shy was a very painful experience for me. I wanted to have a vibrant personality, to fit in, but under all circumstances, I did not feel that I did.

If I were in the company of short people, I felt like I was too tall, or the reverse. If I were in the company of light-skinned people, I felt that my medium brown skin color was too dark. I was not comfortable at all around Caucasians. The fairer an individual's skin color was, the darker mine felt.

Job and I became a perfect match for each other. We became good friends, each of us accepting the other one as he was, not overlooking faults and differences, just never noticing that there were any.

THIRTEEN

May 11, 1999 (Tuesday)

The year is getting away from me, going too fast. Today I taught in the music room of The Friends' school. It is not dark yet but I am tired enough to get in bed. I sat in the recliner in the bedroom and slept, but that wasn't helping me to rest, so I lay across the bed and slept some more. I feel better now. I walked out to the ditch at the edge of our property. I wanted to see what the Township workmen were doing by way of repairing damage they had done to the ditch several years ago.

Daffodils are dead, their once beautiful heads now withered and dark. Peonies will open by the end of the month. Over the years I've noticed that when their time to be in the spotlight comes, it rains, and their large heads, poorly supported by thin stems, droop to the ground.

Seedlings from our silver maple trees cover our front and back yards. The children who used to call the seedlings "helicopters" have grown up and moved away. I hear birds singing summer songs. In the distance is a hoot owl hooting his mournful song. Job is getting more and more forgetful.

May 22, 1999 (Saturday)

My children, and the children of my siblings, are getting together for a First Cousins party. I've been working on a booklet for them. It gives them some background history of their grandparents on my side of the family. I have also written a short profile of each of my ten siblings. I hope the booklet will help them to appreciate each other more as one family unit, even though there are so many of them.

I'm annoyed with Job. He has been rotor-tilling the plot for our vegetable garden. I paid a handyman to have it done, but the workmen repairing our ditch covered up the prepared spot. The ground is very hard and with his bad heart I thought the work of rotor-tilling was too much for him. I told him I would do it, but he has done it himself. Soon I expect him to sit quietly and tell me that he doesn't feel well. He didn't finish mowing the yard. He won't tell me if he thinks it is safe for him to ride the tractor mower.

June 10, 1999 (Thursday)

Yesterday and today we've had wonderful relief from the heat. I've spent a little time today trimming a forsythia bush. I also cut the heads from the peonies. They were no longer beautiful, as the petals had mostly fallen off. On Monday night I saw a firefly flying way up high, the first of the season that I've seen. Carol called. Julian, now four months old, cooed conversation to me. Oh, I am so lonely. I miss Wilma terribly. We were in the drugstore this afternoon and Job had a short-lived incident. His eyes do not look good. Viewing them from behind his corrective lenses, they look overly large, the white of the eye looks sickly white.

He has disconnected the garden hose from the outside spigot, because he declares that that is what he has always done after each use. But that is not true. It stayed outside on the reel all winter. I used it to wash the window screens before I put them up in April. He stores the hose in the shed, which is far enough away from the house that I do not feel up to dragging it out every time I need to use it.

June 13, 1999 (Sunday)

I didn't attend church today. Grace Sands stopped by and picked Job up. I didn't mind not going to church. The time alone gave me a chance to rest mind and body, something I rarely get a chance to do anymore. I put the television on and heard a sermon. A choir sang, "Spirit of the Living God," which was soothing.

Job prepared fish for dinner. I prepared the other dishes. When I walked in the yard I noticed that phlox are peeping open. It is too early for them. It makes it seem like summer is ending when it hasn't even begun. It has been a strange day. Rain

is badly needed and sometimes it seemed cloudy enough to produce some, but none came. At times the sun was out fully. It has
been wonderfully cool and pleasant with no need for air conditioning or fans.

At 9:00 we began watching a movie on television that I suspected would not prove entertaining to Job. Sure enough, only a
little way into the picture he announced that the "picture was not
going anywhere," and he was going to bed. He went into the
bathroom, and presently I heard him crying and muttering to
himself. I was in the living room reading a book. The crying and
muttering went on for a time but I didn't investigate the cause. I
no longer do. I know the cause and there is nothing that I can
do, no matter how hard I try to remove or assuage it. But each
aberrant behavior that he exhibits intrudes itself into a spot of my
upper abdomen, where it lies like an undigested sausage.

Finally, I heard him fluffing up his pillow as he always does
when he is getting into bed. I dread going into the bedroom, not
knowing what I will find there.

June 22, 1999 (Tuesday)
    It is night, past 9:00. For a change Job is in bed early. He
looked so tired. My heart aches for him. We went to fitness center and afterwards to the funeral of the doctor that had been Job's
family doctor since he was a child. The funeral was in the city,
twenty-five miles from our suburban home, and I did not want
to go. With his memory being so poor, I thought Job would have
forgotten about going, and I was not going to remind him, but
he asked what time we would be leaving home to go. Every other
day except Sunday, he asks me over and over what day it is. On
Sundays, he always knows. I told him today that I think he is
selective in what he can and cannot remember. I had planned that
we would go to an Alzheimer's support group meeting tonight,
but our day had been too full and both he and I were too tired
to go.

    June rushing away. Seems it just arrived.

July 11, 1999 (Sunday)
    Tonight I wept because Job is so confused, and I am so lonely.

July 13, 1999 (Tuesday)

Today has been balmy. The temperature is up, but there is no humidity. My great niece Stephanie is visiting with us. She seems comfortable enough with us, but at age 9 she needs entertaining things to do. That presents a problem for me because I am always too tired to take her places that would be fun for her.

Job chipped some small twigs into mulch with his chipper today. He seemed okay, but tonight he looks bewildered. When I ask what is troubling him he says his mind is not working right. This afternoon he was obsessed with the idea that he hadn't had a bowel movement since we came from niece's (my great niece) wedding. That was three days ago. I stopped worrying that he might be right when I remembered very positively that I knew he had had one today. I didn't try to convince him. He is very restless.

July 18, 1999 (Sunday)

Julian is 5 months old today. I called to wish him happy birthday. Carol was feeding him and said he had squash all over himself. As usual, he wanted to play with the telephone cord.

Yesterday the media was filled with the story of John Kennedy, Junior's plane crash. No bodies have been recovered yet, only debris.

There are so many things that Job cannot do anymore, I've suggested that he be responsible for taking his medications for as long as he can handle that task. Last night he had a bout of confusion that reduced him to tears. He couldn't get the pills separated right. Usually if I ask if I can help he decides that he can do it himself, and he has been successful. But he offered no resistance to my helping last night.

He and I are sitting on the patio. I hear cicadas trying to work up a song. Birds are talking quietly.

FOURTEEN

August 10, 1999 (Tuesday)

Oh, what a beautiful morning! When I awoke a cool breeze was coming through the window. I pulled the bedspread up over myself. Lying under it and the sheet, I felt comfortable.

We were to go to the fitness center. I was dressed and Job was getting dressed. I happened to look his way and noticed that he had shorts on and was leaning over the drawer where his T-shirts are kept. He had a T-shirt in hand but seemed confused, and weak. When I asked what his trouble was he mumbled that he was sleepy. He sat in his recliner for a long time but eventually got in bed. I could hear distress in his stomach. That kept up all day. I prepared hot lemon tea and oatmeal for him. He didn't eat much.

Oddly, today is one day short of the day last year when we were at the fitness center and he froze, and we ended up in the hospital emergency room. Later, of course, he was diagnosed with Alzheimer's. Even the weather was just as it has been today.

Dave (my brother) called. His wife died some years ago from Alzheimer's disease. I told him that Job seems to have an obsession with going to the bathroom for bowel movements. He said, "That's the way they do. You never know if there is anything to their complaint or not."

August 11, 1999 (Wednesday)

I expected Job to have some kind of sick spell today, only I thought it would happen while we were marketing, but it happened later. It has been quite warm today, and I guess he was in the sun too long. He was in the bedroom and said he felt faint.

I told him to lie on the bed. He did, and slept for a while. I carried his dinner into the bedroom, but he brought it back to the kitchen to eat. Throughout dinner he alternately ate and sat with his head bowed down. I continued to eat as best I could and acted as if I was not noticing him. I didn't say anything to him. I offered to wash the dishes, but he did them. It's almost 9:00. He seems okay. I am very tired.

August 17, 1999 (Tuesday)
Carol called this morning with a report on Julian's progress. Tomorrow he will be six months old. He is twenty-seven inches long and weighs fourteen pounds. He is crawling. Carol said she left him in his room with his toys and when she went back he was way away from them. The doctor thinks he might walk at nine months.

August is more than half over. Over half the year is gone. Job has had more out-of-breath spells this year than ever before. In fact, he has never had them. He says he is tired. His eyes look sick. Yesterday, he, Amy, and I played Scrabble. Amy was the scorekeeper. She left the room briefly. During the time, I took my turn and asked Job to record my twelve-point score. He didn't trust himself to do it. His mind is so fragile.

I think we are both lonely. He talks to our neighbor whenever he is in his yard, but he hasn't been out much this summer.

HE HAS MOMENTS OF CONFUSION, complains more often of shortness of breath, and feels faint at times, but Job continues to be physically well, as proven by visits to our primary care physician, and his cardiologist. We go places together, and I sometimes leave him at home alone without worrying about whether he will wander away. I have that confidence because at this point I am not yet cognizant that such behavior will probably occur as the disease progresses. He continues to work in our yard, mowing the lawn, putting twigs through his wood chipper making them ready for the compost pile. He never complains about not being allowed to drive, nor does he ask to be driven places. I make an effort to see that we have an outing together every day.

September 27, 1999 (Monday)

Today is my birthday, so I say "Happy birthday to me." It is my seventy -first. Birthdays come hard for me. I do not like the thoughts of getting old. Luckily, today I didn't have time to dwell upon it. I spent the day driving home from Cincinnati. We've been visiting Carol, Aaron, and Julian. He is a dear little fellow. We visited for two weeks, and by the time we left he seemed to recognize us as part of his family.

I did all of the ten hours driving. While we were with Carol, Job was fine. But immediately when we got on the highway he withdrew into his confused state. He wanted to know where we were going. I would tell him that we were on our way home, but moments later he would inquire how long it would be before we got to Carol's house. He also felt that there was a doctor's appointment that he should keep today.

By stopping for only a short rest break, we arrived at home in time for dinner. We stopped at the market and bought something that could be prepared quickly and easily. Job began getting dinner together, but not much time passed before he began to mumble to himself, complaining that he could not locate some item that he needed. He looked tired. I finished getting dinner prepared.

We went into our bedroom, and he just seemed to go to pieces. He was short of breath, he couldn't find anything, he said he was tired. Sleep came soon. During the night he awoke complaining of a severe headache. When I asked him a moment later if his head still hurt, he said no. So, was the headache real or imagined? I don't know. Even when I put my head close to his, I could not hear him breathing. I thought I was losing him.

September 28, 1999 (Tuesday)

At 6:00 on September mornings it is dark. Getting out of bed under those conditions (dark and a bit chilly) was difficult. Yet, it is our day to go to fitness center. After last night's experience, I suggested to Job that he not try to do the full time of exercise on the equipment. He didn't listen to me, and he has been short of breath all day. He is also deep in his funk. He had said that he would prepare the dinner, but by dinnertime I had decided to just leave him alone.

I went down to the laundry room to put in a load of wash. When I came upstairs he was drooping at the kitchen table. He said he was so confused he didn't know what he was doing. Without any words, I cooked dinner.

It is very lonely with just the two of us here. Today I felt myself walking at a slower pace than I did only a few days ago. Can one day into a new birth year make such a difference? I received a number of birthday cards. The one from Job was beautiful.

September 30, 1999 (Thursday)

What a deliciously beautiful day it is. I wish I could hug it to my breast and hold on to it forever. Last night it rained. I don't know when it started. I heard it falling softly when I awoke this morning. It had stopped by the time we left for the fitness center, but dark clouds remained. When we left the fitness center about an hour later, they were breaking down. The dark clouds had disappeared and had been replaced by communities of fluffy white ones that frolicked in various shapes over the blue sky.

We kept an appointment that Job had to get an echocardiogram. He told me that the technician who administered the test gave him a good report: His heart is functioning well. Why, then, does he often complain of shortness of breath? I think it and other complaints are mental.

Carol called. She has returned to work and Julian is adjusting well to his babysitter.

October 5, 1999 (Tuesday)

It is going to be a gloomy day, the kind that seems especially hard on Job, only today he does not have on his dark face of gloom. He hasn't complained of feeling ill. He says he is cold, and has been sitting in our bedroom all day, sleeping most of the time. He has on a long sleeved shirt, a lightweight sweater, and his king robe. The children call it a king robe because it is a really nice one given to him by his co-workers when he had his heart operation nineteen years ago.

Late in the afternoon a little bit of sun peeped out.

October 11, 1999 (Monday)

I've had a busy day. Which of them is not busy? I wanted to

attend the funeral of my classmate and good friend, but it was far away, and I was not familiar with the route that I would need to use to get to the funeral parlor.

The weather is beautiful. There are no clouds in the sky. It has been warm but Job has sat in our bedroom all afternoon dressed as if it is wintertime. He has the portable heater on and the door closed. The room is like a sauna.

Today I dug up and replanted a sapling oak tree that for the past two years has been growing to close to the house. I wanted to save it because over the past thirty-seven years we've lost several large ones. I hope this one survives.

October 19, 1999 (Tuesday)

It is just after 9:00 PM. I have just gotten into bed. Job went earlier but he is not asleep. The day has been bright and crisp. At times the wind blew vigorously. Crabapples from the decorative tree on our front lawn rained down.

We kept our appointment with the urologist. Job has had periodic checkups since his prostate surgery eight years ago. When his examination was over the doctor came to the door (unusual for him) and said we needn't see him again until this time next year. That was really funny, because as we were driving to the office I remarked to Job that maybe we should stop our visits to the urologist. Am I prophetic or what?

The nurse, from his chart, I guess, noticed that Job was taking Aricept.

"But he looks all right," she said, "maybe the Aricept is helping."

I don't think so, but most of the time he does seem perfectly normal. At other times, UGGH! Tonight, for instance, he ate ice cream for dessert at dinnertime. Less than an hour later we came into the bedroom to watch the news and he ate another bowlful. Still later he was preparing to have a third serving, not realizing that he had already had some twice before. It's too much to write about. It is exasperating.

Before coming to bed I looked out of the window on the still night. Lights in a few houses were on. I saw a star in the clear, night sky. I didn't hear the sound from it, but I saw the lights from an airplane that was winging its way to somewhere.

FIFTEEN

❦

November 1, 1999 (Monday)

We've just returned from a trip to Cincinnati visiting Carol. Aaron was away on a business trip. Being with our little grandson was such fun. He is sweet, and playful. This time we flew out and back. Even so, getting reoriented to being at home proved difficult for Job.

He went into the bathroom to get washed. I thought he was okay, but I found him in the living room still in pajamas. When I asked him why he said he couldn't find any of his belongings, not his toothbrush, nor his travel kit, nor any of his clothes—it was so unnerving.

I went to substitute teach in a school. When I came home he had mowed the lawn, and had also started dinner. After dinner I cleaned up the kitchen.

I do not often go out after dark, but tonight I needed a few items from the supermarket and went to get them. Driving to and from the market, memories of the times we went grocery shopping at night came back to me. The children were little. We would wait until Job got hone from work and he and I and the children would go to the A&P supermarket. The store has been gone from our area for many years.

Things seem so different now. Just that week spent with Carol seems to have put us into another phase of our lives. Job's and my togetherness is not really togetherness. A big wall separates us and only I can see it. When Job was well, just being together was all we needed for happiness. We fulfilled each other's needs. Now I have no one to talk to.

November 11, 1999 (Thursday)

It is bright and sunny again today but lots chillier than the past two days. I helped in the nursery school today. The drive to school was beautiful with colorful fall foliage. I find myself hurrying home to be with Job. I see, but do not want to see that his mind is deteriorating. Today we went to the fitness center before I left for school. When I did leave he was just starting to eat a bowl of cereal. The rest of his breakfast was already prepared. Marty had lots of other help. So I played my two songs and left.

Job was still in his workout clothes, which was unusual for him. But he had no recollection of having been to exercise, nor did he remember that he had already eaten breakfast. I gently coaxed him into getting dressed.

Last night he talked to Amy. I heard him telling her that he had started to compost his garden plot for next year as this would probably be his last garden. How I hope it is not. It is so sad. I try to remember how it once was with us but a lump, not big enough to push the tears out (oh, how I wish it would) gets in the way of my remembering.

November 22, 1999 (Monday)

On this date thirty-six years ago President John Kennedy was assassinated. I was pregnant with Carol and had stopped work, waiting for her birth, which would be in December. Our nation and nations around the world were sad.

This day has been gloomy. I've spent it cooking things that I can put in the freezer for Thanksgiving dinner. We are not having company. Only Job and I will be at home. I persuaded Carol that she should not try to travel. Amy will have dinner with her in-laws so that she can have Christmas dinner with us.

It is unusually warm for this time of year. Yesterday and today the temperature is in the 60's.

I've wrapped some Christmas gifts, although it doesn't seem like Christmas. Job has been gloomy and weepy for most of the day. I go on with my life.

November 30, 1999 (Tuesday)

It is early morning this last day of November 1999. We've been for our exercise, had breakfast, and washed and put away the dishes. All other chores are done. It is cold today but not as arctic as TV announcers would have you believe. There is bright sunshine and floating white clouds. The house is quiet except for the radio. It is tuned to the classical music station.

The stereo hasn't been played for a long time. I think Job has forgotten how to operate it, and I never knew how to, although he tried to show me how many times. I didn't try hard to understand, because I counted on him to do things for me. Now, he can't do things, and I don't know how.

December 8, 1999 (Wednesday)

Wow, the month is well underway and I've not recorded anything. In a way that's good, because if there were negative behaviors that I should have written about Job, I would have.

We've just returned from a visit with Amy and James. They are still in their apartment but they have purchased a house. We didn't have time to drive out to see it.

I've been busy, baking cakes, pies, and cookies. Wreaths for the windows have been lying on the dining room table for a week. I thought Job would put them up for me but he hasn't done so. He hasn't mentioned Christmas at all. It is sad. He used to get so excited about it.

As I was coming in the front door this afternoon I noticed that my snapdragons are still blooming! And last week I noticed that daffodils for spring 2000 are about 2 inches above ground. The weather has been that warm. Still, we have also had some fairly cold days.

Fly away December. Come along, Christmas. It doesn't seem like Christmas. This year I am not even buying a poinsettia, something I have done for many, many years. I will put up a tiny tree, because Carol asked me to.

December 17, 1999 (Friday)

I awoke to hear Job sobbing. When I asked him what was the matter he said his mind wasn't working right. I didn't react, did not offer sympathy, didn't say anything. I knew that he was feeling sorry for himself because I was annoyed with him yesterday for trying to repair a part of the refrigerator that was broken. I knew that he could not repair what was wrong and asked him to PLEASE just leave it alone. It is not a new behavior that when he is angry with himself he takes his frustration out on me.

Hey, all by myself I figured out how to work the stereo. We listened to "Messiah" twice. Now I know how to play the CD part of the stereo and how to set the clock on the VCR. Wow. In the afternoon we went to the store and Job bought Julian a toy. I've not bothered him about getting gifts for anyone else.

December 22, 1999 (Wednesday)

Our dental appointments for today have been rescheduled. I wish they hadn't been so that we could have gone and gotten the dread job over with. We went to the supermarket but were home in time for the noon news. There's lots of talk about terrorist threats against Americans at home and around the world.

Today is the first day of winter. In three days another Christmas will have come. My house is decorated. I set the tree up and trimmed it except for the lights and the angel. Amy will put the angel on when she arrives. Seeing that I was not going to ask him to do it, Job added lights to the other decorations on the tree.

This morning a few snowflakes fell. It is cold, but not very. The house is quiet. Hoping for Christmas music I had turned the radio on. When none was played, I turned it off.

Soon I will take Job to get a haircut. He seems well enough today. Yesterday he was bad. He couldn't get anything right. I went to bed and fell asleep only to be awakened, I think, by his muttering to himself. I thought he said, "I hope I can keep my sanity until Christmas." When I questioned him for an accurate account of what he said, he said he was talking to God. Yesterday he seemed so normal, like he was a perfect specimen of mental acuity. It's like that. If one day he is good, as seasons follow each other in an orderly pattern, I can count on the next day to be positively hellish.

December 24, 1999 (Christmas Eve)

We had picked Lois up from the city yesterday. On this Christmas Eve night she and I stayed at home while Amy, Job, Carol, Aaron and Julian went to Christmas Eve service at church. Lutherans have more services at Christmas time than any other denomination I know of. It was not a part of my family's tradition to attend church service on Christmas Eve. We lived in the rural South without the convenience of modern methods of travel. We did well to get to church on Sundays, especially during the winter months. So, none of my siblings nor I enter into these seasonal religious observances that call for attendance at other than regular Sunday service. It was probably different with Job. He was born in suburban Pennsylvania and that's where he grew up.

After dinner and all had returned from church we sat and watched Julian play. James was not feeling well and went to bed early.

December 25, 1999 (Christmas Day)

Christmas belonged to Julian this year. It has been fun watching him enjoy the toys he received. James has been ill all day and has spent most of it making a valiant effort to join the rest of us, but losing, has stayed in the bedroom lying down.

December 30, 1999 (Thursday)

Fast away the Old Year passes. The weather for this time of the year is still warm. The temperature today climbed to 50 plus degrees. As I entered our front door I noticed a single, yellow snapdragon clinging to life. We are going to Maryland to ring in the New Year with Amy.

James was admitted to the hospital early Monday morning with the diagnosis that he has suffered a very mild, heart incident. He is to be catheterized to determine the extent of damage to his heart. His illness has cast a psychological pall over all of us. Carol, Aaron, and the baby will visit James in the hospital then leave there and head back to Ohio. I feel weak and nervous. I guess I am concerned about Amy and James—married only a year and now he has had a heart attack.

December 31, 1999 (Friday)

How strange it seems. Tonight is the last time forever that I will use the 1900 numbers to mark a New Year. Tomorrow, if I live to see the day, I will experience the year 2000 come in. All of my lifetime, and the lifetime of all my siblings, I have written 1900, and now that is about to change.

Carol and Job are preparing some make-ahead meals for Amy.

I've helped by folding and pressing some of James' myriad shirts. Newspersons have reported that in Times Square, New York people have been gathering since 7:00 to usher in the New Year.

Have I made New Year's resolutions? Yes, to write in my journal every single day.

SIXTEEN

With her (his) first hello
She (he) gave a meaning to this empty world of mine.
There'd never be another love, another time
She (he) came into my life and made living fine.
She (he) fills my heart

THAT'S HOW IT WAS, OUR BEING TOGETHER. I noticed that before he trusted himself to speak words to me he seemed to turn them over in his mind first, as if weighing them to see—to see what? If they would come out properly structured grammatically? To see if the topic was something that I would approve of? I never knew, but there was no mistaking the brief hesitancy and intake of breath before he articulated his thoughts.

Our courtship continued in a way that I am sure is quite different from how young couples do things today. During the late 1980's when I was in my sixties, I worked with a young man who was single. One Friday when it was almost time to leave work for the weekend, I said to the young man, "So, John, is tonight date night?"

"Date night?" he countered earnestly, "What's that?"

I explained that that was what we called going out together in my day. The whole act of dating was different then, at least for Job and me, and I strongly suspect for others of our generation as well.

He would come by public transportation from his suburban home to mine in the city. Sometimes we would go to a movie. Eventually he held my hand. His fingers were long, and thin, but they felt strong. As our relationship grew, he graduated to letting his arm rest on my shoulders during the movie. I was pretty uncomfortable with that but did not strenuously resist, didn't resist at all as a matter of fact. Dating was practically a new experience for me, and I did not want to appear awkward, besides, I rather liked it.

Between dates we wrote each other long love letters, and called each other later to discuss the contents of the letters by telephone. On one date he arrived at my home with a single rose, of the genre Peace, which he had grown in his flower garden. It was a beautiful flower. Even now the image of its pinkish yellow color is etched vividly in my memory.

Gardening was an interest that he developed prior to being drafted for military service just as the Second World War was almost over. Everyone was encouraged in those days to plant a Victory Garden if it was possible to do so. Where I lived in West Philadelphia no spot of concrete was willing to yield its place to a spot of earth sufficiently large to support vegetation. Job's yard at his home in Ardmore was large and fertile enough that he could and did grow both flowers and vegetables.

Planting a "Victory" Garden was his exercise in patriotism until after his graduation from High School in June of 1945. His tour in the army lasted for a little over a year, as the war was, or soon would be, over by the time he entered the service. He was assigned to the Army band, where he used his skill of playing the clarinet. He had begun the study of that instrument in Junior High school, which is today's equivalent of Middle School.

By extending his studies of the clarinet he had honed his skills enough with the instrument that he was accepted as a musician with the Main Line Symphony Orchestra. While his brothers had taken advantage of the GI Bill to attend universities, Job had used the money to attend music school.

Just being a member of such a prestigious organization as the Main Line Symphony Orchestra I thought was wonderful beyond words, but Job admitted modestly that someone other than he occupied First Chair.

When the orchestra performed at one of the Main Line Middle Schools, I went with him and sat in the audience. When there was no score for his instrument in a composition, he joined me. Having him beside me gave me a wonderful sense of pride. I felt very fortunate to have him as both friend and suitor.

SEVENTEEN

NOTHER YEAR HAS ENDED. We have known for a year that Job has a disease that is terrible in the devastation that it inflicts on its host. And yet, not until I turn the pages of my journal do I, realize how stealthily and ambitiously the disease has engaged in the work of destroying the brain of a once brilliant mind, as well undermining the love and beautiful relationship that had existed between a happily married couple.

January 1, 2000 (Saturday–New Year's Day)
I must get accustomed to writing 2000. When news commentators or other speakers with access to public forums spoke of the year 2000 five or ten years ago, that time seemed so remote, so far away. Now it is here, and is half an hour old. We sat up and watched the celebrations of countries around the world.

We are still visiting Amy. We've been to the hospital to visit James. I cooked dinner.

January 2, 2000 (Sunday)
The day is beautiful; the temperature climbed to 60 degrees.

January 3, 2000 (Monday)
We came home from visiting Amy in Maryland today.

January 6, 2000 (Thursday)
Since Job is unable to help me make decisions, I must read everything myself and make the best decisions I can. That's what I've been doing today—reading, making decisions, and filing papers away. It is so wearying.

Also, his state of being confused has begun for the year, I guess. When he came out of the bathroom he was still in pajamas and didn't know what he was to do next. Often he resists my help. Today he didn't. When we came from the fitness center he seemed better, almost himself

January 7, 2000 (Friday)
Job has done an excellent job of getting dinner together. It is almost like pre-Alzheimer's days, when I relaxed while he prepared dinner. He read the paper and was able to discuss some news items with me. He also read some from the book about exercising the brain that Amy gave him.

January 13, 2000 (Thursday)
Dinner is over and Job is washing up the few dishes that remained to be cleaned and put away. He helped get dinner together by preparing the fish and watching to see when it was done. I had prepared the other dinner dishes early in the afternoon. I find it is better to do it that way, otherwise, he starts hounding me and looking nervously at his watch around 2:00 or 2:30. We never eat before 5:00.

He is so restless, poor man. Poor me also. I am grateful to God that he is still with me. Still, dealing with his behavior is very trying. He is company for me, but there is nothing of our pre-1998 life left except our existence.

January 17, 2000 (Monday)
Since I learned how to operate it I've been putting CD's in the stereo regularly. Job never, ever bothers to. He seems to not think about things that he at one time liked. He used to put garlic on his ground turkey breakfast patty. Now, he doesn't. Tonight we played our game called "Upwards." But before we finish any game, he loses interest.

January 19, 2000 (Wednesday)
It hasn't been as cold today as it was yesterday. I've done quite a bit of running around, to the supermarket, to the Dollar Store, to Wrightstown. I carried my lunch with me to Wrightstown and sat down and ate with Marty, Joan, and Sue. We would be hav-

ing soup and a salad for dinner. I had told Job the menu several times. I ordered a cake from the discount store. I was not too tired to get the dinner together, but I was weary from all the running around I'd done. Job asked what he could do to help get dinner ready and I suggested that he make the salad. He makes delicious salads. I sat in our bedroom resting, but something told me to check to see how he was making out with the salad. I found him just wandering around in the kitchen. I reminded him gently that he was making the salad. He sat down and cried. I went back into the bedroom, but eventually I went out and made the salad. He has been quiet all evening. We're in bed now and he is sleeping.

January 24, 2000 (Monday)

The snow is melting rapidly, although in this state and others deaths have resulted from icy road conditions. It is sad. I pray that our children will get to and from work safely. Indeed, My prayers include all people, but I suspect that God does not appreciate my usurping his role of calling to Eternity whomever he wants, whenever he wants them.

Especially I pray that little Julian will not be hurt in an accident.

Today it has been almost balmy when compared to last week's frigid temperature. It only reached 40 degrees, but it seemed much warmer.

I had bought some items for Lois and carried them to her. Driving along the Schuylkill River, I noticed that it is still frozen over. But I could discern some thin patches of ice, signaling that thawing is occurring.

We had leftovers for dinner. It took him a long time to do it, but Job got dinner together. Tonight, though, he's in a crying mood. Oh, how I hate that.

I was playing the piano. He was in our bedroom watching TV. When I thought I heard him moving about I went in to check. He was dressed for bed but agitated. He said nothing worked right for him. I assumed that he meant that he couldn't get a clear picture on any of the TV channels. Sometimes he pushes a wrong button on the remote and things go whacky. I have no clue as to how to make it right. I just keep pushing buttons until a picture shows up.

We talked about our children, and he talked about himself.

When I was riding home from my visit with Lois I started to feel sad about him, and about Wilma. I never dreamt that my life would come to this. When you're young, you don't.

January 30, 2000 (Sunday)

We made the 9:00 service. It's nice to get in from church and have some free day left. I rested for a while before preparing dinner. I wanted to fall asleep but couldn't. Job got angry with me and went to bed at 8:30. By 11:00 he was up and dressed, thinking it was another day. I left him alone until he started to take his morning medicine. I couldn't let him do that. Even so, he was angry with me again and threw the box of pills into my lap.

I must look for the next support group at the fitness center so that I can attend. He went back to bed but was up and dressed again by 2:00. I asked him to please not go out. He yelled at me and asked if I thought he was crazy. He argued that he was only going out to bring in the paper. I assured him that the paper would not have been delivered yet, that it was too early.

He did take his morning medicine and sat, fully dressed, in the living room for the rest of the night. I didn't fall asleep until after 3:00. He came back to bed at ten minutes before six.

January 31, 2000 (Monday)

He was up by 8:00. That's the time I got up. He has slept a lot today. It is now 8:30 PM, the same time that he went to bed last night, and it looks like he is getting ready to go at the same time tonight as well.

I know that he took his medication at the wrong time, and I worried about that, but there is nothing I can do. Is he getting worse? Will he from this point on be like an infant, confusing night and day? He has hardly uttered a word to me all day. I think he knows that he has acted badly, but as has been the case all along, he'll make no hint of it.

Yesterday a light snow fell that is now crusted with ice. I cleaned off the cars and shoveled some of the driveway. Mr. Armino was doing a little shoveling, clearing a path for the mailman, he said.

February 1, 2000 (Tuesday)

I feel teary today. I don't know of any one reason why. It's probably because of a combination of things. I talked to Carol tonight then Job spoke with her. She seemed pretty upbeat when she and I talked, but with him she seemed disturbed about something. Job told me later that she is concerned about the plane trips that she must take for her job. There was a plane crash yesterday. Hearing of her concern made me tense.

Amy and James have become homeowners. They signed the agreement yesterday. How I wish I could protect my children from all life's hurts.

After fitness center Job helped me clean our bedroom. He seems a little better, a tiny, tiny, bit better.

Snow is melting slowly.

February 2, 2000 (Wednesday)

Snow still covers the landscape. Streets are pretty much dry and free of ice. Marty called for me to come and play the piano for her morning class. I had lunch with the staff. My playing went well. Carol called. Julian wasn't feeling well yesterday, but he is better today.

Diane called to tell me that presidential candidate Senator John McCain was in Clinton, South Carolina campaigning. Wow! Imagine! A presidential hopeful in the little town where I was born? My father would have said, "Who wooda thought it."

Days go by fast. I have no energy or ambition to do anything more with my life than to cook, take care of Job, and keep the house tidy. I do not write except in my journal. I do not practice the piano.

February 4, 2000 (Friday)

We didn't do much today except run a few errands. In the afternoon we played a game of Scrabble. I won the game, but Job played well. It was a good friendly game until the very end. He had one tile left, an "I." He put it on the board and I said it wasn't really a word. He got very angry and said he thought I was wrong. We ate dinner in silence.

February 8, 2000 (Tuesday)

How did I let the other days get away from me, the days when I wrote nothing down? Maybe nothing happened worth noting. Maybe I was too tired. Emotionally, or physically? Could be either one. Job is getting more and more fractious. I don't know what to say to him or when to say it.

Twice in the past week he has gotten angry with me when I tried to offer help. Once was when I saw a single pill on the shelf where he keeps his medications. I tried to show him the right bottle to put it into. He said, angrily, "Maybe I should just kill myself." It was upsetting. I didn't want him to even entertain such a thought.

Last night I asked him if killing himself was what he wanted to do. He replied, again angrily, "No, but you always think I can't do anything right." Today, no matter what he did, I left him alone. It's 8:00 and already he is in bed. I hope he doesn't get up and wander about.

February 13, 2000 (Sunday)

We went to early service, so the day has seemed especially long. I didn't need to cook dinner, just heated up frozen ones that I had prepared earlier. During this long day, not much conversation has passed between the two of us. It's like the two people that we were are dead and different people now inhabit our bodies.

February 29, 2000 (Tuesday)

Today is our first day of being at home in a while. We spent two weeks in Cincinnati with Carol. Julian celebrated his first birthday while we were there. We had left our car at the airport. We picked it up and drove from there to Maryland to visit Amy. It is the first time we have seen their new home. It is beautiful.

We got home yesterday, but I had all the usual Monday things to do—laundry and sundry mundane tasks.

Early in the morning we exercised at the fitness center. I went to Wrightstown to play for afternoon class. I can still leave Job alone but I often take him along with me just for the ride. Today was such a time. The day has been beautiful but a little chilly. The weatherman has just said that the temperature is 57 degrees and may go to 60 tomorrow.

I can't put my finger on anything specific that happened today, but something did cause me to wonder how Job can seem so "all right" when he is away from home and so miserable when he is here.

February 3, 2000 (Friday)
We went to the Senior Citizen Center to get our income tax prepared. We were surprised to see our friend Clay Banks there. He has prepared our income tax for us for several years, but last year he wasn't at the Center to volunteer. We understood that he was not well. He has had problems that have left him unable to walk without the aid of a cane. Still, I have never seen him look at all depressed.

I wish Job could have taken an example from Clay and continued to try to do things.

March 6, 2000 (Monday)
Up early. Busy day. I had bought Julian a little suit that I hope he will wear to church Easter Sunday. I packed it and mailed it at the post office. While out, I stopped in Kohl's Department Store to see if they have a pillow that I can use to sit up in bed and read with. I had to throw my other one out. Maybe we only need one. We both used to sit up in bed and read, now I am the only one who does.

For the past couple of weeks Job has gone to bed around 7:30. He has slept for most of this day but already, at 8:00, he is in bed and has turned over for sleeping. In less time than an hour he will get up and dress for going to the fitness center. I will try to keep him from taking the medication that he should take tomorrow morning. I don't know where our lives are headed.

March 13, 2000 (Monday)
We had an appointment with Dr. Howard today. We hadn't seen him since last September. The neurologist reported that Job was down from twenty-three things remembered to nineteen. Today he was down to thirteen things remembered. Oh, well, I guess that means he's sinking fast. The doctor said that when he first saw Job in 1996 he was remembering twenty-seven out of thirty words quoted. He is going to increase his Aricept dosage

from 5 to 10mgs, and is also going to try giving him vitamin E.

The sun is shining but it is chilly. Job took a walk around our yard. I hear him talking to our neighbor. That's good.

March 14, 2000 (Tuesday)

Only one day left until the middle of the month. I've been uptight all day. Last night I got very upset with Job and he with me over the pill thing. I had told him some time ago that I wanted him to continue doing that task all for as long as he is able to. Well, he really isn't able to anymore. I need to monitor his medication taking and he doesn't want me to. Last night he didn't take any of his pills although all are critical to his health: Aricept for Alzheimer's, Isosorbide for his heart, and Atacand for blood pressure.

He wouldn't go with me to the fitness center, but he did take a walk around the yard. I was pleased that he stopped to chat with our other next-door neighbor.

We went to the post office and to the bank. It has been warmer today than yesterday. I walked to the back of the yard to look at the tiny crocuses. Daffodils are budding. I need to begin cleaning the house thoroughly. We used to call it "spring cleaning." Does anyone do that anymore, or am I dating myself? Anyway, I have no energy for doing anything. All of my energy is expended on trying to attend to Job.

March 15, 2000 (Wednesday)

Went to Wrightstown today and played for the afternoon class. They are still studying dinosaurs and enjoy singing "The Dinosaur Song." I stayed at school longer than I had planned because a little boy with the biggest bluest eyes imaginable asked me to sit at the Play Dough table with him and make spaghetti-o's, and I did.

We ate dinner at The Old Mill Inn. That is, we started dinner. Halfway through the meal Job didn't feel well, so we boxed things up and came home.

I know that his condition is getting worse. It is not noticeable in a big way, that is, outsiders would probably not notice. But he gets facts mixed up. When I came from Wrightown yesterday I noticed that he had worked some in his garden plot. He asked me if I would take him to the nursery to buy tomato plants. "Isn't it a bit early for that?" I asked. He said no, that he always had tried to get his tomato plants in the ground by the first or second week of March.

Nothing I could say (although I didn't try very hard) would convince him otherwise. I knew emphatically that he had always said that he would not put tomato plants in the ground before May fifteenth, because after that date our region would probably be free of further frosts.

March 16, 2000 (Thursday)

Job had an appointment with our Primary Care doctor. Dr. Miles is so nice. We couldn't ask for a more caring physician. Since Job's memory has been bad I have been sitting in the examining room with him in case the doctor needs to ask me questions. Physically Job is fine. His heart and lungs were good, the doctor said.

We did little things when we came home. I raked leaves from three flowerbeds. Then, I relaxed for a while. Dinner would be the leftovers from our unfinished meal at the Old Mill Inn last night.

At bedtime I noticed that Job had put one Aricept and two vitamin E capsules into the little cup I set out for his medications. He still had a Lescol capsule that he should have taken at dinner, but he said he had taken all of the pills that he was due to take, and the ones in the cup were those that he would take tomorrow. I am fairly certain that he had not taken the ones that he should have. He gets so angry when I question him. Should I bother to do so? I don't know.

March 18, 2000 (Saturday)

I went to a funeral in the city and left Job at home alone. I often leave him alone if I am called to substitute at school, or if Marty calls me to come to Wrightstown. I always worry when I leave him alone, wondering whether he will be all right. I generally check on him by telephone. Even in the summer when trees are thick with leaves I can see our backyard from the street. As I rode along I saw him working in the garden and breathed a sigh of relief that he was okay.

March 19, 2000 (Sunday)

Every Sunday morning Job asks me what time church service starts. Last night I put a note on the bedside calendar that I had given him for Christmas noting that the early service starts at 9:00, the later one at 10:15.

I knew it would happen. This morning he kept lifting his head and looking at the clock and the note. At twenty past eight he asked, "Do you think we can make the early service?" I can't win. We, of course, went to the 10:15 service.

I talked by telephone to Carol and heard Julian say words. His vocabulary now includes, "hello," "dog," "book," and more.

March 21, 2000 (Tuesday)

This first day of spring has been cold and rainy. I don't know why Job was reluctant to go the fitness center. We went, and he interacted pleasantly with his "buddies." Most of the men there have known him for many years. They don't know yet that he is not well. Thank goodness for people who do not treat him as someone who has the plague. I, perhaps unfairly, think I detect that attitude in some church members.

We went to the new IHOP for breakfast. The interior is beautiful, but I didn't enjoy the food. At home I had a lot of housework to do. Some Job could have helped with, but he sat downstairs in the family room with his head down. We both had been there to watch a video that we rented on Saturday. The film had been rewound incorrectly, and I discovered that it was not going to work. It made him angry that I took the film with me. I knew that if I left it with him he would try to make it work and possibly ruin it in the process. Sometimes I must take matters into my own hands. This was such a time.

Eventually his mood changed, and after I told him what we would have for dinner, he prepared it.

March 23, 2000 (Thursday)

I am so tired I can barely move. Yet, soon I must start dinner. Exercising at the fitness center is the cause of my tiredness. I've only done a few outside errands. One was to go to the card store and buy a birthday card for Job. His birthday is tomorrow. I've ordered a cake from Country Manor Bakery.

March 24, 2000 (Friday)

He's seventy-three today. I gave him his card early in the day. A separate one from Julian and Carol came in today's mail. Carol called in the afternoon to wish him Happy Birthday. He and I went to dinner at The Old Mill Inn. We used the gift certificate that Amy had given us at Christmas. From dinner we went to a movie and saw "The Cider House Rules." At home we ate birthday cake and ice cream.

March 27, 2000 (Monday)

Today I went to a support group meeting. It was held in the same complex as the fitness center. Only four people were there, two women other than myself, and one man. All of us were caregivers of Alzheimer's spouses. The accounts the others gave of their loved one's behaviors were so depressing, I'm not sure that I will attend other meetings.

One woman reported that her husband stands in front of the commode but urinates on the floor. The other woman said her husband slipped off in the car and went to the store. Luckily, he got home safely. The man was reluctant to talk about his wife in front of other women.

I think I have it bad. Their cases are much worse. Maybe Job will not get to that stage. I am comforted by that thought

Forsythia bushes are in full color. Daffodils are beautiful and prolific. The day was clear. At night it rained. I fell asleep listening to the sound of it gently pattering down to the earth.

Carol called. She has taught Julian to growl like a lion. He gave a mighty growl for me over the telephone. Carol said that it is okay for us to come and visit them in May.

EIGHTEEN

April 27, 2000 (Thursday)

Tuesday night Job complained of having a headache. He didn't actually voice a complaint, just was very quiet, and frequently removed his eyeglasses and held his head. He seemed to have a cold, but although he blew his nose often, it appeared not to be a productive effort. When I would ask if he wanted to visit the doctor's office he would give his usual non-committal answer.

I thought the headache might be signaling a stroke and insisted that we go to the doctor. Our regular doctor was not on duty. The attending physician asked him if he had a cold. "No," he said, but added, "well, maybe a little in my chest."

I couldn't believe he was saying that. Why had he held his head and complained of a headache? Was that an imagined pain? The female doctor checked his blood pressure and felt that a stroke was not threatening. When we returned home I asked if his headache was gone, and after two days of complaining about it, he said, Yes." Still, he continued the behavior that caused us to visit the doctor in the first place.

The weather is still dreary. Sometimes it rains. Often it is just cloudy.

May 9, 2000 (Tuesday)

Ignoring warnings for elderly people, and those with respiratory problems to avoid being outside in 90+ degree weather, yesterday Job mowed our entire three-quarter acre yard, pulled weeds, and dug up daylilies for replanting. Today, he didn't feel up to going to the fitness center. Every time he tried to do anything he would get dizzy and disoriented.

When I got home from the fitness center he was eating breakfast. He finished, and I helped him into the bedroom, where he sat in his recliner. Less than two hours later, he went into the kitchen and began preparing another breakfast. He became dizzy again and went back into the bedroom and got into bed. At 2:00 he got dressed and went into the kitchen to prepare still another breakfast.

I realized that something was desperately wrong and suspected that it was related to his having stayed in the sun too long. Quickly I got out our Home Emergency book and looked up "heatstroke." He had all the symptoms of this condition that were listed. I followed the book's instructions for treating the problem, and eventually he was all right. I believe, however, that had I not reacted as I did, he would have died. The book listed death as a possible result.

May 11, 2000 (Thursday)

Fitness center day again. We both went together. Job seems fine—his old self, hardheaded, and raising his voice to assert that he is right when usually he is wrong. I don't argue. I am too tired.

On Tuesday when he was very sick and I was so tired from walking back and forth to administer to him, I tried to imagine what life without him would be like. When after all I had done to make him better he was so ungrateful, I reasoned that being alone might not be so bad. I would use the time alone to allow my body, mind, and soul to heal from the pain that I am suffering.

May 31, 2000 (Wednesday)

May stayed around a long time, yet, looking back, it slipped hurriedly away. At the beginning of the month I was busy, substitute teaching at Buckingham, going to Wrightstown to play for morning and afternoon classes, and preparing for our trip to Cincinnati.

We were there until the twenty-fifth. We came home and went right away to Maryland to visit Amy and James. Carol, Aaron, and Julian came to visit them also while we were there, and we had a lovely time.

Tears welled up when I left the children on Monday, and all day yesterday I felt sad and alone, with tears standing at the threshold but never springing forth. My stomach quivers with nervousness.

The day was gray early this morning. Maybe that is what got Job in a crying mood. Gray days do seem awfully hard on him. He got up in a confused state. He had put his razor in his little travel kit where it is not usually kept. I knew where it probably was and got out of bed and found it for him. By this time he was totally confused. He had put on his under garments but didn't know what to do next. I got out a shirt and trousers for him.

Preparing his own breakfast is something that he can still do, but I still set everything out for him. Still, he is quiet, moody, and crying. I'm leaving him alone. I have problems of my own, not the least of which is him.

There is yard work in abundance that needs doing, but on this perfect day for outdoor work, Job has made no attempt to do any. Oh, well.

June 1, 2000 (Thursday)

A new month has begun. Our calendars have been turned reflecting the change. Turning them is my job. In his present condition it's like Job is in a time warp. The matter of time simply escapes him.

Since we've been home from our trips he seems more "out of it" than before. Noticing the changes that are occurring, my stomach knots up. I want to weep, but tears bunch up as a lump in my throat. Lois telephoned tonight, but no one else. I want to call the children, not to complain about their father, but to hear their voices, which are a comfort to me. I am resisting the urge to call them.

I am in the kitchen where the only sound comes from the humming of the refrigerator. Outside, birds chirp merrily. Today it has been hot and humid. When we came in from the fitness center there was a call on our answering machine. It was from a school, wanting me to substitute. Mentally, I had planned to spend the day reading, resting, and having the day, as much as is possible under the circumstances, to myself. I returned the call to the school and went to work.

June 2, 2000 (Friday)

The temperature is way up again. I had bought plants from the nursery and invited Job to help set them out. We would do the work while it was early, and while we could work in a shaded area. He chose not to do that but to weed whack instead. Even to do that, he began after the heat and humidity was beyond where he should be doing that kind of activity. I went out to where he could hear me and advised him that if he allowed himself to get sick with heat exhaustion as he did before, he was on his own, as I was not physically able to do again what it takes to bring him around.

I sometimes think he refuses to listen to my advice because it is too much like loosing control of taking charge of his own actions. Today, wonder of wonders, he did stop what he was doing, and went next door to our neighbor's and the two sat under a big shade tree chatting.

June 3, 2000 (Saturday)

What a difference a day makes. The small amount of rain that fell last night cooled things down tremendously. Both Job and I were able to work in the yard. It was cool enough that he needed a lightweight jacket. I didn't. I finished setting out my plants. Job commented that my flower garden looks nice. I only bother to garden because he doesn't, although he used to. He mowed the lawn and weed whacked. Our yard is so beautiful. Roses, peonies, and flags are in bloom. Deep purple flags bloom by pink peonies. Way in the back of the yard white peonies are in bloom, and all around the circle where our above ground pool used to be, are roses in different shades of color.

June 13, 2000 (Tuesday)

Soon it will be the middle of the month, then, July 4, a time that, for me, is the beginning of the end of summer. Soon, it will be the Twenty-First Century. It is night, a hard time for me. I try to think of things to do that will hold Job's interest. I have books that I would like to read, but he doesn't try to read books anymore. He looks over the newspaper but I know that he is not reading—or at least he does not comprehend what he is reading.

What a pity that television fare is so poor. We enjoy watching Seinfield, but that show is over and nothing else appeals to us. I suggested that we play a game of Scrabble. He said, "OK," but continues to keep looking at his watch and consulting the TV listings. He has put the TV off but just sits, looking glum. He has made no effort to take me up on the offer to play Scrabble.

June 16, 2000 (Friday)

Yesterday was cold, gray, and dreary, but it was not cold enough for Job to put a turtleneck sweater over his shirt. He continues to be quiet and uncommunicative, as if his mind is as dull as the weather. In the afternoon he seemed better and went next door to talk with our neighbor. Mr. Armino was riding his tractor mower, but he stopped to talk. How things change! Mr. Armino used to walk over to our yard to chat with Job and Job would just keep doing whatever job he was engaged in. I've told Mr. Armino about Job's condition and he says he understands.

June 20, 2000 (Tuesday)

Summer is to begin at 10:00 PM they say. By that time it will have been preceded by a beautiful summer day that has been golden, with blue sky decorated by large, shapeless clouds.

I had been after Job to weed whack the portion of ditch abutting Monroe's fence that he can't clear with the tractor mower. He has insisted that the Township is going to "fix it." He didn't believe me when I informed him that the Township had finished their work on our property. The uncut part spoils the beauty of the rest of our yard, so I tried using a scythe to clear the long stretch, but the job was too difficult for me. I think Mr. Marino convinced him that nothing more would be done by the Township.

In the afternoon I went out alone, but I always find myself hurrying home to see if Job is all right.

June 26, 2000 (Monday)

Job was up early and readied himself for going to the fitness center. When I told him that our day is tomorrow he went into the living room, sat in a chair, and slept until after the noon hour. Even after that long spell of sleeping, he slept some more, until late afternoon. It was frightening, but he said he felt okay.

June 27, 2000 (Tuesday)

We always eat breakfast after we've done our exercising. Even though I set everything out for him, getting his breakfast together still confuses him. Maybe I should just do it myself, but for as long as he can, I want him to continue to do for himself, hoping that will help preserve his mental acuity.

I set his place at the table, but he spends lots more time rearranging a job that I feel that I have done well. It exasperates me that he must straighten the place mat, and adjust, (over and over again) the silverware.

Again today, he slept a lot. Why? Is his condition worsening? He talked well enough to Carol last night. He rarely talks to me.

June 29, 2000 (Thursday)

It is almost 7:30 PM. I am siting outside at the old, round, picnic table. Job mowed the lawn today and occasionally I look up to enjoy the clear, fresh look of it. Phlox have started to bloom. Our black-eyed Susans are in bloom all over the place, and on the bank, daylilies are beginning to open.

Job seems lots better today. He has been quiet all week, not talking, just sitting in a chair in the living room either sleeping or feigning reading the paper. He came out to the patio and sat for a moment then decided that he should mow the lawn, but the lawn is already freshly mowed. He just seems not to know what to do to keep himself busy.

I spoke to him about his behavior, telling him that I am afraid that he has completely withdrawn from reality, and that puttering about in the yard is something that he once enjoyed doing. I didn't get a response. He merely went back inside.

NINETEEN

❦

July 4, 2000 (Tuesday)

I can only hope that somewhere, someone had a happy Fourth of July, with beach parties, picnics—anything that brought them joy. Our day was sad. Nothing different happened. Is there anything that I could have done to make it different? I don't think so. I have no ingredients, no tools, no materials, nothing to make happiness happen.

At breakfast, Job sat at the table looking as if he were exhausted. I asked if he wanted me to prepare his breakfast. He said, no, that he would do it, and he did.

If I sit on the patio he will come out briefly, but frequently pops up and down and goes inside. In and out, in and out, he goes like a waiter serving patrons on a restaurant's patio. Late in the afternoon Amy called. How pleasant it was to hear her voice.

July 10, 2000 (Monday)

Amy and James had come up from Maryland and spent the weekend with us. When someone other than the two of us is in the house it is ever so much more pleasant for me. It is as if a great pressure is lifted from me. Amy went to church with him. He likes to go to church and I take him, but there are times when I go but do not really want to.

Today we went to the mall and I did a bit of shopping. Mostly, I go places so that Job has an outing. We were home by 5:00. After dinner, while Job washed the dishes, I worked in the yard. Lately he has set the table for breakfast when he finishes the dinner dishes.

This evening when he finished the dishes he came outside

and we sat on the patio, although he followed his pattern of get-ting up and down frequently to go inside. Then, the strangest thing happened. I thought I heard him say something to me. I didn't hear clearly, and he didn't repeat what he had said, so I went to investigate.

I found him in the kitchen eating a bowl of cereal. When I asked why, he said he was eating his breakfast. Oh, God, have You forsaken me? Have You forsaken him who in his faithfulness to You is so like your servant Job of ancient times? For though You slay this present day Job, I know he will trust in You as long as his he is in command of his faculties. The disease is getting worse.

July 13, 2000 (Thursday)

Job had his regular check-up with Dr. Miles. His heart, lungs, and blood pressure are good. I told the doctor about the frequent trips to the bathroom. He suggested that we reduce the dosage of Aricept from 10mgs to 5mgs. After all, he said, no one knows whether the medication helps or not. I told him that I would like Job to continue taking it.

July 17, 2000 (Monday)

Carol is coming to visit. We went to the toy store to buy toys for Julian to play with when he comes.

After dinner we sat on the patio and I heard cicadas sing a short chorus. I've heard them only once before this season. That was when the weather was warmer a few weeks ago.

July 19, 2000 (Wednesday)

I was very, very sad today because snatches of scenes of past years kept flashing across my memory screen. A mere glimpse into the past, and then the scene would disappear.

We went to the bank. Job suffered a bout of confusion that was of short duration. Most of the day went well, but he cannot remember anything from one second to the next.

July 20, 2000 (Thursday)

He suffered more confusion today. At the fitness center he insisted that he worked out on the rower first. Which piece of equipment he does first doesn't matter, it is the tenacity with which he holds on to an incorrect fact that reveals the severity of his illness.

After breakfast he went out to inspect the garden. When he came in he sat looking forlornly in a living room chair. I asked him if he was okay. He said he felt all right, but his mind wasn't right. I am concerned about whether reducing the dosage of medicine was the right thing to do. I don't know.

I suggested that we go for a ride. I try so hard to keep him busy, keep his mind working, even though I feel that I am fighting a losing battle. We went to Kohl's and to lunch afterwards. Tonight I insisted on helping him get his medications together. He hated it and did his best not to cooperate, but rightly or wrongly I stood my ground. He is so ill.

July 21, 2000 (Friday)

It has been another beautiful July day, with large white clouds hanging from a blue, blue sky.

I have noticed that every time Job goes to take something from his wallet, all the little cards fall out of it—bank card, Social Security card, insurance card, everything. Each time this happens he opines that he must buy a new wallet. I always remind him that Amy gave him a new one for Christmas, 1998. Today he left the wallet on his dresser while he was working in the yard and I took the opportunity to transfer the contents from the old wallet to the new one. He hasn't (and won't) noticed the change, and I am more comfortable knowing that he will not lose a valuable item such as his Social Security or bank card. I've thrown the old wallet away.

July 31, 2000 (Monday)

Today is a big letdown after the flurry of activity of the past several days. We were in South Carolina attending a family reunion. Being "back home" is always fun for me. Job is a Pennsylvanian, so he usually feels a little lost in the unfamiliar surroundings, and in the company of people that are, for the most part, strangers to him.

I am now back to doing mundane things, and Job has settled into his quiet/angry mood. The out of doors has the look of

August. Crabapple leaves are turning brown and falling to the ground. Apples from our non-decorative trees are also falling. Job picked up a basketful. Tomorrow I may make applesauce and can or freeze it. Carol and Julian are coming for a visit tomorrow.

August 21, 2000 (Monday)

It is the birthday of one of my nephews. Richard's, I think. On Saturday we went to the city and visited Lois for about an hour. Later we ate dinner at a new restaurant that recently opened up in our area. It's pretty nice. The weather was a perfect summer day, but Job was all bundled up in a winter turtleneck, a jacket, and a cap suitable for winter weather.

August is waning. It doesn't seem that it was so long ago that at this time of year we would be taking our girls back to college.

Sunday we attended the early service at the Lutheran church.

Back to today's happenings. I've spent a good portion of it outside enjoying the delicious summer weather. Job, on the other hand, has sat in our bedroom with the windows closed, the space heater with its two heat control positions on, and he's wearing a turtleneck sweater plus the jacket to his workout suit. I think he is just trying to push my buttons, but I don't comment about it.

My neighbor asked me if Job talks about dying. She says her husband does. She wonders if he is getting Alzheimer's because he repeats the same thing over and over just as Job does. Mister Armani has always been very neighborly. He and Mrs. Armani are a little older than Job and I. I hope he is only suffering from the forgetfulness that comes with aging and not with Alzheimer's disease.

August 22, 2000 (Tuesday)

He is just being obstinate. I know it. It is not hot enough to turn the air conditioning on. Besides I prefer not to use it unless it becomes absolutely necessary. I do like to keep the windows and doors open to keep the house comfortable. Job wore only a tee shirt to the fitness center, but when he came home he put on his winter turtleneck. When he sat down to breakfast he noticed that the window was open, so he put his workout jacket on and put the hood up! I ignored him. I must remember to confiscate that turtleneck and put it away until winter. The temperature is in the 80's. When he went outside and was talking with Mr. Armani he took the workout jacket off but kept on the turtleneck. He always closes the doors when I open them. I open them back up.

August 24, 2000 (Thursday)

Yesterday he had a spell of faintness. When he thought he was better he stood up but made no steps to go forward. I suggested that he sit back down, but he didn't move to do that either. I hope his brain is not shutting down completely. Today he is okay and doesn't remember anything of yesterday's incident at all.

August 27, 2000 (Sunday)

One month from today I will turn seventy-two-years-old. I still remember things that happened when I was five years old: Mom and I visited Aunt Mary in Lansing, Michigan. We traveled by Greyhound bus. We had to sit on the very back seat because we were black. At least I was black. Mom was much lighter but that didn't matter.

When I was eleven years old I went back to South Carolina from Philadelphia where I had stayed with my older sister for several years attending school. I remember being happy to be back in South Carolina with my parents and other siblings.

I remember when I turned twenty-one and decided that I wouldn't bother to vote because I didn't think my vote counted. At age twenty-eight I got married. I remember being forty and thinking that I didn't feel old.

August 28, 2000 (Monday)

I saw the name of one of Job's high school classmates in the obituary column of today's paper. He had Alzheimer's, wandered away from home and fell into a lake and drowned. Is that something that I must look forward to happening to Job?

September 11, 2000 (Monday)

Time flies when one day of uninteresting happenings blends in with another day of the same. I keep the house tidy and take care of Job. Probably if there were more stimulating things to be done, I would be too tired to participate in doing them.

Today, Job fell off the toilet seat. Why would that happen? Did he fall asleep or become momentarily unconscious? I heard a loud thump and rushed to see what was the matter. I found him lying on the bathroom floor. He lay there for some time before he was able to get up. He was not unconscious when I got to where he was lying. I kept talking to him. By the time he finished getting dressed for the day and came to breakfast, he had no memory of the fall. He was not hurt by the fall but it left an ugly bruise on his right thigh.

It is almost the middle of September, but at nighttime I still hear the chirping of crickets, the cooler weather making their chorus sound weaker than when the weather is hot.

A SCAN THROUGH JOURNAL ENTRIES REVEALS that no behaviors significant enough to report about have been recorded. During this interim there have been difficult days however. I know that difficult days will be my constant companion for the rest of our lives together. Often there are disagreements about his medications that disturb me. Also, there is the difficulty of getting him to shower and change his underwear daily. In time I will learn to "pick my battles," engaging in the absolutely necessary ones and ignoring those that are not. I am about a year away from knowing that this is what I must do in order to preserve my health and my sanity.

TWENTY

November 7, 2000 (Tuesday-Election Day)

We've been to Cincinnati again. Little Julian is a powerful drawing card to that area. We had a great time playing with him. Julian loves his "Bepop," his understanding of the pronunciation of "grandpop." Whatever he was playing he wanted "Bepop" to join in, but Job mostly sat on the end of the couch and watched. So, it was I who pulled the little doggie with the short string around his neck while Julian pulled Dino the dinosaur with the longer string.

We were both tired when we got in from the airport at 8:00 last night, and when Job suggested that we not unpack our bags until morning I readily agreed. This agreement, however, led to the first time I completely lost my patience with him and became hysterical with frustration.

There were medications that needed to be taken at bedtime. When I looked for them in the bag that I had packed them in, they were not there. Had I left them in Ohio? I was sure not because I had checked that bag specifically before leaving. When I asked Job about them he had no idea where they were. I began to scream and cry uncontrollably. The hysteria lasted for a full five minutes, with me trying as hard as I could to get myself under control, but I simply could not. I can only liken my behavior to an airplane that has touched down to a scheduled landing with the intent of staying down, but without intent, takes off again in flight.

Should I have reacted as I did? No, but as I said, it was an involuntary reaction caused by one too many frustrations. I would try to put his medicines in places where he could not find them, but he would find them. I tried to keep my medicine hidden, but he would find that as well—and take it if I were not looking. So, especially when traveling, I was careful to keep the medications in a bag that I would carry. My frustration arose from knowing that he had deliberately transferred them to a different piece of luggage as a signal that he was in control of his life.

November 15, 2000 (Wednesday)
    Today is the halfway mark of the month. Time goes by so quickly. Job's and my relationship hasn't been good lately, but it is getting better. I try to be patient, and in my mind I succeed. It is hard for me to accept that at times he is perfectly rational while at other times he seems deliberately obdurate.

December 29, 2000 (Friday)
    Watching the year wind down leaves me feeling sad and lonely. I slept late. Job brought the paper in and I skimmed news items, focusing more on the editorials and letters to the editor. I particularly like reading items dealing with political currents.
    I've done a few errands. Job has had some malady all day that he thinks is indigestion. Seems indigestion wouldn't last all day. He has been quite restless. Once he went down to the basement and was there for a long time. When I called down to ask what he was doing, as happens often, he didn't answer. I went down to check on him. He was looking in a closet that he doesn't usually bother with, since he has no need to.
    "What are you looking for?" I asked him.
    "I thought I had some Christmas gifts in here," he answered. For the past couple of years he has shown no interest in buying gifts. None that he would have received would have ended up in the closet that he was looking in. I am sure that he just needs something to do but he will not act upon anything that I suggest.
    Since I have been caretaker to him, I often ponder my fate in old age. Who will care for me? Like most parents, I do not want to be a burden to our children.

December 30, 2000 (Saturday)
    Only one day of the year 2000 left. At this time last year we were in Maryland visiting Amy and James. James had had a mild

heart attack. Today we had our first big snowstorm of the season.

I have not done much except try to read with understanding two annuity contracts that I have. I have also made cookies. Job has slept a lot. I asked him why he did not try to engage himself in some activity. He hasn't done so. He has only wandered aim-lessly about on the unfinished side of our basement.

December 31, 2000 (Sunday)

Another year is ending. It is foolish to do so, but I can't help trying to envision what the New Year will bring. It is afternoon, almost 4:00. We didn't attend church, no reason why, I just elect-ed not to go.

Job went outside and cleared the cars of snow. Sometime dur-ing the morning he asked me what day it was. I told him Sunday but that we were not going to church. Oddly, he didn't complain. Lawns in our development are blanketed with snow. I took the camera outside and Job took a picture of me in the snow, then I took one of him.

I rented videos so that we will have something to do to cel-ebrate this New Year's Eve. At midnight Amy will call. Carol may call also.

ANOTHER YEAR IS DAWNING. Unlike the ones I have already written about, for the upcoming year I do not need to turn the pages of my journal to know what lies ahead. The year's collective events are etched in my memory as solidly as the faces of the four pres-idents carved in stone on Mount Rushmore.

Still, I will turn the pages one by one, as they apply to the encroachment of the disease that is changing my husband into someone whom I hardly know, so that you may see the deadly Alzheimer's beast at work. It begins to attack more swiftly now, like a conveyance, unchecked by bridle or brakes, descending a hill.

TWENTY-ONE

She (he) fills my heart
With very special things, with angel songs
With wild imaginings
She (he) fills my soul
With so much love that anywhere I go
I'm never lonely
With her (him) along who could be lonely?

O
N OUR SECOND DATE he proposed to me. I sensed his inter-
nal preparation for asking me to marry him, even as I
prayed silently that he would not do so. I liked being
with him, and I presumed that how I felt about him was because
I was in love with him. But was it love or "just a second-hand
emotion?" How could I be sure? I needed desperately to be sure—
against the warning of my father who told me that his sister was
forty years old when she let some man "fool" her. To hear that
from my father was very embarrassing. I did not want to be
fooled, nor did I want any encumbrances that would preclude my
attaining the goals I had set for myself.

So, when Job finally articulated his proposal I told him that
I really liked him well enough to accept, but I would need some
time to think about it, to sort out some things about marriage and
life in general that I needed to find answers to.

We visited each other's churches. I liked going to his because
it was in the suburbs, was small, and had a sunny, beautiful interior, whereas mine in the city was large, old, the exterior was of
dark, gray, stone, and sunlight did not readily penetrate the spacious sanctuary.

I liked sitting beside him in the church pew. Enough hymnals were available so that each of us could have held our own, but we didn't, preferring instead to share, allowing for an occasional touching of hands. Hearing him singing, I noticed that his voice range was bass, whereas because of his slight build I would have imagined it to be tenor.

He was of such a slight build that never in his wildest dreams could he have aspired to be a football player. He stood just a head above my five foot four inch height, which may have disqualified him as a basketball hopeful as well. But in high school he did run track he told me, admitting that in that sport he would never have rivaled the celebrated Jesse Owens. It was a sport that he was comfortable with, he said, and he enjoyed participating in it.

Despite not having a large frame, his clothes fit perfectly, as if they were tailor-made for him, indeed, some were. Those that were not were altered to a proper fit, so that he always looked clean-cut and neat, with no bagginess or sagging in the seat of his trousers, and with no ill fitting of his suit jackets.

As a couple we were a contrast in skin coloring. Mine was medium to dark brown, while he was light skinned but not fair. He looked good in any color shirt that he chose to wear except yellow. That pastel accentuated negatively his coloring, which to me seemed a cross between an apricot and an anemic pumpkin skin. His eyes, I had ample opportunity to observe, were light brown.

On dates he took me to the nicest places: to the theatre, to orchestral concerts, to the best restaurants. We continued to be involved in activities of our respective churches.

Not until I had a daughter to reach the dating age did I appreciate why my parents were so concerned about our being together so much for such an extended period of time. I knew that he was always a perfect gentleman. In all instances his first consideration was my well-being.

His one vice that I knew of was smoking cigarettes. This would be a probable contributing cause to the heart attack he suffered later, but it was not out of the norm of our day. It was a habit with many young men and some women. He didn't indulge in drinking alcoholic beverages, and with but one exception, he neither cursed nor swore.

The one exception to cursing happened after we had been married for some years. Carol, our oldest daughter was little but was old enough to realize that daddy had "said a curse," and that saying such a word was out of character for him.

We had been on vacation and were returning using a toll route. Job had the required change necessary to toss into a basket and continue to drive through. Other cars were behind us. When one of his coins missed the basket Job said, spontaneously, "Oh, hell." And just as spontaneously Carol quietly remarked in total disbelief, "Daddy said a curse."

Enough years have passed that Carol no longer remembers the event. I remember because of how precious it was to me that she considered daddy to be in all things above reproach. Considering the situation, I would not have accused him of being out of character for saying the offending word. I had no dream that the day would come when that language and worse would be directed towards me.

TWENTY-TWO

January 1, 2001 (Monday)

Amy, I am beginning the New Year by using the nice journal that you gave me as a present for Christmas, 1999. It is much better than the composition books that I have used for so many years.

It is ten minutes before 1:00. I had to sit up alone to welcome the New Year. I had rented two videos and made popcorn, and even bought Raisinettes for Daddy, but he went to bed before "Touched By an Angel" went off. I'm surprised that he awoke at midnight to take your call.

Our development was quiet at midnight, no fireworks or noisemakers as in years past. I guess like you and Carol, the young people who would make merry have all grown up and moved away.

Snow is still on the ground but it doesn't present a problem for driving, so we went about doing errands during the day. For no special reason, we went to Willow Grove Mall. I stopped in Barnes & Noble and bought the book "A Fly Went By." Carol wanted a copy for Julian. I still have most of the books from when you girls were little, but that one had been handled so much it was falling apart.

It is night now. With this day I began my journey towards my seventy-third birthday. I wish I were younger. There are things in life that I wanted to do that are not done yet. I don't feel old, but I am.

January 2, 2001 (Tuesday)

It seems everyone knows that I like to keep journals. My hairdresser gave me a small one for Christmas. Tonight I offered it to

Job to use to write down anything of the day's activities that he could remember, no matter how insignificant it seemed to him. He wouldn't do it, just went to bed at 8:00.

He had borrowed a book from the library. I brought it to him but he showed no interest in reading, even when I suggested that he read a page and I read a page. I try all sorts of things to do to keep him mentally stimulated.

Yesterday, I tried getting him to recall incidents that happened during the four years we dated. He said he remembered nothing about that period of our relationship and very little—if anything—of the forty-three years we've been married.

January 4, 2001 (Thursday)

Job has been pleasant all day, but for the past two days he has refused to engage in any activity. He doesn't even attempt to read the newspaper. I expect him to have one of his infrequent bowel accidents in bed because he became confused about his medications and his pajamas and wouldn't allow me to help him set things right.

I didn't make any New Year's resolutions, but I am settling into it with the resolve to just try to take each day as it comes.

I called Carol tonight. She said Julian asks about all of us: Aunt Amy, Uncle James, Aunt Lois, Grandmom, and Grandpop.

January 6, 2001 (Saturday)

We didn't go to the fitness center because I felt the weather was too bad. Later in the day we went to Circuit City. Carol had given us a gift certificate so that we could purchase a new TV for our bedroom.

On my way out, I slipped on ice and fell flat on my back. I didn't think I was badly hurt. We went on to the store. Job and I were playing a game of Scrabble later and my hand began to pain so much I had to get into bed. It was only 6:00. Job was playing poorly anyway, so I stopped the game.

I keep wondering how long Job will have some mental capacity left. There are times when he seems reasonably okay. At other times he doesn't seem to connect at all. Wintertime seems hard on him, but then last summer was pretty bad as well. I am tired. My heart seems tired.

January 8, 2001 (Monday)

I slept until 8:oo, which for me is late. Instead of feeling rested, however, I feel sluggish. The sky is overcast. I think I heard
rain falling against the window glass.

We went to our safe deposit box and I brought everything
that was in it home to check out.

At night we played a game of Scrabble. I won the game. It
was Job's idea that we play a second one. We had not begun to
play before he was totally confused and sat with his head down,
and a countenance of midnight dark. What, in so short an interval, could have caused such black despair?

"What's wrong," I asked.

"I'm just confused," was his reply.

"OK," I said, "we won't play anymore."

Even with me checking his medications, sometimes at the end
of the day things are not right. What should I do? I don't want
to make him feel useless by taking away everything that he has
always done for himself.

I am so tired. I am getting sick. I have no aches or pains, but
I can feel the sickness coming. I feel worn out. My heart is heavy.
I can feel it thumping hard in my chest and back. I'm afraid I am
going to have to tell the children how I feel. I am afraid that I
am going to have a stroke.

January 9, 2001 (Tuesday)

Job was so good today it is frightening, because I have
observed that there is a definite pattern to his behavior. If one
day he causes me no grief, the next day he is sure to be impossible to live with. I've come to apply this little nursery rhyme to
define his fluctuating temperament:

There was a little girl
And she wore a little curl
Right in the middle of her forehead
When she was good she was very, very good
But when she was bad, she was horrid.

I spent the day sorting out papers and writing in a composition book what they are about, and where they can be found. I'll
do the same for Job's when there's time. If my mind starts to go

(sometimes I feel that it has already) I want our children to know where all of our important documents are.

It is still cold. I fell on the ice again today. For the rest of the winter I am going to wear boots. I can't afford to break any bones.

January 10, 2001 (Wednesday)

Went to school and played my two songs for the nursery school children. We went back to Circuit City and bought a TV set. Now there's the job of reading directions for setting it up. How I miss Job's ability to do those things now. He was the one who always read directions for operating appliances then patiently explained them to me.

For some years now I have been reading the obituary columns in the newspaper, looking for names of classmates from my 1947 high school graduating class. Today the name of one of Job's friends was listed. It was noted that he had been in a nursing home and had died from complications of Alzheimer's.

It is 10:00 at night. I hear the drone of an airplane. Where could it be going? Job's day was not as bad as I thought it might be.

January 11, 2001 (Thursday)

Amy, I really like having this journal. I keep it right by my bedside and that helps me remember to write. Of course I still must make time for doing that. Often, even though I remember, I am too tired to do anything but crawl into bed.

Snow has melted enough that I can see the entire compost pile as well as around tree stumps. There is a sizeable clearing between Monroe's fence and the ditch part of our yard.

At the fitness center we saw some of the old-timers. Since Christmas we've gone later because of weather conditions, so we've missed seeing the early birds—the ones who habitually arrive by the time the Center opens at six.

I made cookies today and encouraged Job to help. The most recent material on Alzheimer's that I've received suggests letting the impaired person help with tasks. With that in mind I asked him to take the washed clothes from the washing machine and hang them on the lines in the basement. Things were going well, then I reminded him to take the two pills that are due to be taken at lunchtime.

I noticed that the pill for cholesterol was still in his pillbox. That was okay. It wasn't due until suppertime. But then I noticed that other pills were not in the box at all.

I questioned the discrepancy, because I do try very hard to see that he takes his medications. When I asked how that happened he went into his spiel of, "I know what I'm doing. You think I don't know anything. You just want to treat me like I'm a child or something."

At night he spends from half an hour to forty-five minutes and more getting his medications into the little pill organizer that I bought for him. During this time he opens and closes the medicine bottles many, many times. He flips open the compartments of the pill box many, many times. It drives me crazy. Once a pill is out of the container, he loses track of which pill is which and tries to determine by color or size the right one to put into a compartment.

When I can't stand it any longer, I get out of bed and try to help him. This makes him angry and he ends up throwing the medicine bottles (closed, thank God) at me. It took a while, and added another layer of stress to the knot in my stomach, but I learned to just leave him alone. Always, however, after I am sure he is fast asleep, I take medicines and pillbox into the bathroom and sort them out, so I knew that every morning all medications are properly distributed.

When I ask him if he would like me to ask Dr. Miles if I should take charge of dispensing the medications he gets darkly quiet and angry and says he has no thoughts about it.

I'm desperately afraid that I will have a stroke. To whom can I go for answers? I must hurry and get our papers in order.

January 13, 2001 (Saturday)

I went to Staples and made photocopies of important papers that I feel our children should have. On Monday I will mail both girls a package of copies.

Job is still able to get dinner together sometime. He did today. We both went down to the rec. room to watch TV. I set his bedtime medicine out before going downstairs. He decided to come upstairs but said he would be back down. I figured out that he was up to something. Sure enough, when I came up he had taken his nighttime medication as well as the ones that had been prepared for morning, including two isosorbide pills that should be taken one three times a day.

"That's it," I told him. "From now on I am taking charge of administering your medicines." I must buy a lock box. I'll get one from Office Max.

January 14, 2001 (Sunday)

I bought the lock box, and I've told Job that there are to be no questions about it, I am giving him his medications.

Having done that, tonight I feel more relaxed, as if one burden of concern has melted away from the great pile that crowded my stomach. Something else will spring up, I know. What? For instance there is this constant itching that continues over most of my body. Lately I've felt it on one side of my face, and in my head. Is it a precursor to another attack of sarcoidosis? That's always in the back of my mind. If I get sick who will take care of Job?

Although tonight I feel weepy, I do not feel keyed up.

Today was overcast but it was warm and comfortable.

January 15, 2001 (Monday)

I've done a lot of chores in a relaxed way today. Job has not objected to my giving him his medications. I put mine in the lock box also, as he has not been above taking one of my Evista pills. That's all the medicine I take except for a multivitamin and an 81mg aspirin.

January 17, 2001 (Wednesday)

I still feel relaxed, but am I possibly developing Alzheimer's? Sometimes I forget what day it is.

I've been telling Carol that I feel as if I am getting ill. She has contacted via computer a nursing agency that I should contact for relief from my caregiving. A nurse came to see me today. She said that I had done absolutely the right thing by putting the medicines under lock and key. I was glad that I had already figured that one out for myself. I feel good about having such prescience, if that is indeed what it was.

Job has been good all week.

January 19, 2001 (Friday)

I went to Wrightstown today but wasn't there very long. The visiting nurse supervisor came to our house today. I filled out papers so that if I need their services I'm registered.

Today is the last day of President Clinton's presidency. I admired his academic brilliance. I wish I had never learned of his character flaw. That was something that I felt I didn't need to know about. I also admired Jesse Jackson's brilliance and am disappointed that he also has a flawed character. I do not feel the need to judge either man.

In the distance I hear a fire engine.

Job is wandering around. I know he is looking for his medicine bottles. I suspect that he searched for them while I was at Wrightstown. He is in bed now, breathing heavily, not saying anything, as he does when he is angry or upset about something.

January 21, 2001 (Sunday)

I am so pleased with Job's attitude of late. Today he prepared dinner all by himself. He still does things that annoy me. For instance, he will see my perfectly empty, dirty dinner plate, already placed by the sink for washing, and ask me if I'm finished with it. He will call with the same question even if I am in another room. When putting the dishes away he puts everything in the wrong place, but I am overcome with love for him when I see him trying so hard to do the right thing.

January 22, 2001 (Monday)

Night is approaching, but daylight lasted for a long time. Even now at almost 6:00 there is a wee bit left. Job has come into the bedroom from the kitchen and closed the draperies, so I will not see when darkness has fully come.

We will watch the news on the Public Broadcasting channel. Before we retire to bed we will read a few Psalms. I suggested that we do that in order to keep him familiar with words. I will read a Psalm then he will read one. Sometimes we read several a night. They're beautiful. I hope it helps.

January 24, 2001 (Wednesday)

Job seems to be doing really well these days. I know there is no reversal for his condition, but these interludes of near normal-cy are precious. Three times this week he has actually showered instead of "getting washed up" in the bathroom sink. We contin-ue to read from the Psalms. For the past few days we have worked a little on playing two-hand piano. The pieces are sim-ple. We bought the music book to encourage Carol to practice with Amy when they were younger.

He plays the primo part, which has fewer notes. So far he has played only the right hand part. When he tries to combine that with the left hand he gets confused. Given time, though, I think he will master it.

January 30, 2001 (Tuesday)
    Job has acted strangely all day.

January 31, 2001 (Wednesday)
    Today has been beautiful. It has been warm. In the morning I went to Wrightstown. In the afternoon we food shopped. I feel myself getting tired again, and my stomach is knotting up. I haven't had outside help yet. I must call the agency and have them send someone next month.

January 5, 2001 (Monday)
    When I looked out of the kitchen window after breakfast I noticed that large, watery flakes of snow had combined with already falling rain. The temperature was 38 degrees, and the snowflakes so watery I thought there would be no snow accu-mulation. I was wrong. Fifteen inches fell in Quakertown. With weather as a worry bone, it dominated the day's news, interrupt-ing other programs. Schools were let out at 12:30. Power lines came down. Traffic was snarled on most routes, city and subur-ban. Snow fell all day.

We read our Psalms, but Job did not want to practice the piano. I didn't either.

January 6, 2001 (Tuesday)
    After yesterday's snowfall, today was clean up time. I went out to shovel our driveway. Soon Job came out and said he would do it. I reminded him that since his heart attack twenty years ago

he wasn't to shovel, especially the wet, heavy kind of snow to be dealt with. He went back inside and sat and sulked for the better part of the day. Late in the afternoon he announced that he was "Going out for some fresh air." I knew what that meant. When I looked out he had shoveled the entire patio plus a path from the patio to the shed. I am angry. I probably will have to call the doctor tonight. I hate having to make the determination of when to call. It is particularly annoying when I know that the call is being made because of Job's stubbornness.

The temperature was up nicely, providing the warmth necessary to melt the snow considerably.

On days such as this one I visualize the route we used take when visiting Wilma and Steven in New York. I visualize the mountains we would see as we drove along route eighty-one, then on up New York Route 41A along the Finger Lakes. At times the calm, blue water of the lakes was visible. Along other stretches houses or trees obstruct the view. I miss making those trips up to Auburn. I miss Wilma.

February 7, 2001 (Wednesday)

Job had an appointment with the endodontist. With that done, I spent the day puttering about, reading things that must be read, doing little things that eventually must be done.

February 9, 2001 (Friday)

Today is my free day. There is absolutely nothing that must be done. I played well at Wrightstown. When the children went off to their "work," I came home. We went to the Senior Citizens' Center to file our taxes for the year 2000. Too many people were ahead of us, so we came home. For an outing, we went to the drugstore.

Job still walks all stooped over because of the extensive snow shoveling on Tuesday. He looks quite haggard. I am offering no sympathy, although I hate to see him suffer.

February 10, 2001 (Saturday)

Job's back is still out, so we didn't go to the fitness center. I had things to take to the city for Lois. He went with me. On the drive down he had a short "out of it" spell. He tried to get some words out but couldn't get them together. I turned the heat off and opened the window a crack. The incident lasted no more than a minute.

February 11, 2001 (Sunday)

Our only outing on this sunny, slightly cold day was to attend church. When he gets up from a sitting position Job still assumes a stooped position—from the snow shoveling, I guess. Some of his behaviors make it quite evident that he has some dementia. He doesn't seem mentally stable. I hope it all passes soon.

February 15, 2001 (Thursday)

My appointment with Dr. Miles was for 10:00. I was on time and went right into the examining room. I sat there draped in my paper covering for the better part of an hour. He must have been running late. I don't usually have to wait that long.

I was given a clean bill of health. I thought it best to mention to the doctor how my heart felt. I told him that it feels tired and heavy. He said it is probably broken. He knows how I've had to endure Job's heart attack and by-pass surgery, as well as a prostate operation with its attendant consequences. And now this.

Today has been cloudy and dreary. Spring is on its way, however. This morning I heard an owl's sad lament.

February 16, 2001 (Friday)

Our visit to the Norman's for Job's haircut was our only outing for the day.

Doris was not at home. We chatted briefly with Richard, both friend and barber, then came home and had dinner. After dinner I looked for the tray for the toaster oven broiler/baking tray. Job had cleaned up the dishes and misplaced the tray. When I discovered it missing I searched and searched all areas of the kitchen without finding it. It is so frustrating. He had no idea at all of what I was looking for.

February 17, 2001 (Saturday)

After fitness center I spent more time searching for the broiler/baking tray. I went back over all the places I had already searched, living room, dining area, upstairs, downstairs, the outside garbage receptacle, the compost pile. I was worn out from hours of searching as well as from frustration. Finally, quite by accident, I spotted the tray blending in with the partitions of the stainless steel dish drain.

February 19, 2001 (Monday)
Spent the day trying to understand papers that I had requested from the Bucks County Agency on Aging. I don't know what to do. Also, as a Veteran Job is entitled to a reduced cost for drugs through their plan. I began filling out papers to take advantage of that.

February 21, 2001 (Wednesday)
I heard birds talking when I went out to bring in the paper. I recognized the raucous caw of crows but not the voices of birds with softer voices.

Carol called and I talked to Julian. She told him to say, "I'm being difficult," and he said quite clearly, "I'm being difficult." How I would love to see him, to hold him and let him fall asleep in my lap. What a wonderful diversion that would be from my current daily routine.

February 23, 2001 (Friday)
Today is our forty-fourth wedding anniversary. If we make it to fifty I'm sure Job, if alive, won't know it. It is good that our anniversary is today. We have tickets to the Philadelphia Orchestra matinee. They are season tickets but we can pretend that we bought them to celebrate our special day.

We received cards from friends. There was one for me from Job. He had spent a lot of time selecting it. Still, the one he bought read, "Happy Birthday." I crossed out the "Birthday" and inserted "Anniversary."

We ate dinner in town so we didn't get home until 5:30. Something, perhaps the glass of wine I had with dinner, made me ill and I went directly to bed. When he came to bed later, Job tossed and turned with such restlessness I had to get out of bed. I sat in his recliner and slept until he fell asleep. Such was our Happy Anniversary. I hadn't given it much thought anyway. My thoughts are absorbed in the here and now.

February 24, 2001 (Saturday)

He doesn't even remember that yesterday was our anniversary.

February 26, 2001 (Monday)

By six o'clock Job was up and dressed for going to the fitness center. When he discovered that this is not our day to go, he had something like a quiet fit. Over his tee shirt and sport shirt he put on a heavy sweater. On top of that he put on his "king" robe. He has turned the thermostat up to eighty degrees. The portable heater is on. Even so he has sat shivering in his recliner all morning. He has offered no hint of what his problem is. I guess he is waiting for me to ask him. I am not going to.

It has been a lovely day. I went to the post office. In the afternoon I walked to the back of our yard. Daffodils are shooting up fast. Buds on the silver maple trees are beginning to turn red.

We received a package from our girls today—an anniversary gift. They are wonderful daughters. I am so alone.

February 27, 2001 (Tuesday)

Looking out of the window at the fitness center I saw a robin. I got really excited about that and called to others near me to come have a look. For most of the day I've felt relaxed, a rare occurrence. At times I become anxious thinking about the coming of spring and summer when Job is less likely to spend his time indoors. Will he be able to use the tractor mower? And suppose when operating it he forgets how to reverse? What will happen? I shudder to think about it.

February 28, 2001 (Wednesday)

This last day of the month is bright and sunny, but it belies the outside temperature, which is quite cold. I went to Wrightstown. The time it takes to get there seem longer and longer each time I drive out. Of course, I'm not as young as I was eleven years ago when I started going out there.

Carol called tonight. She said Julian is a handful and that when the new baby comes and we come out to see her, she's going to send him home with me. She's kidding, of course. She loves that little boy.

Every morning when I wake up I feel very tired. Probably it

is because I don't conserve steps as much as I should when doing things around the house. Seems like my eyes are getting dimmer, but I still only need to wear glasses for reading.

March 1, 2001 (Thursday)

I'm waiting for a call from Aaron to say that Carol has had their new baby. He called earlier to tell us that she has gone to the hospital, her water has broken, and she is having contractions. It is 9:00 and he hasn't called back. We'll have to wait a while longer, I guess. I may fall asleep.

March 2, 2001 (Friday)

We have a new grandchild, a little girl. Her name is Alana Nicole. Aaron didn't call last night. That's a man for you. How could he know how anxious his wife's mother (and father) would be about the health of mother and baby? I've spoken with Carol. She and baby are fine. I wanted to talk to Julian but he is still with the friend who is keeping him for Carol.

Job and I went to the mall and bought things for the new baby. I intended to mail them today, but when I got home from shopping I was too tired.

March 5, 2001 (Monday)

Snow and icy weather kept us from going out today. Late in the afternoon I cleaned snow and ice from the car. I also made a cake to take with us when we fly out to see the baby.

I can see, but try not to, that Job is getting worse. Sometimes I feel very sorry for him because he appears to be trying so hard to do things right, but things turn out all wrong for him.

Today is gray. I thought things were going well. We had decided not to go to the fitness center. The streets didn't look bad, but they didn't look good either. After breakfast I missed Job. I found him in the living room looking very, very sad! When I asked his what was the matter he said, "I don't know why you don't want to be with me anymore."

"What're you talking about?" I asked him. My heart sank. I had no idea of the origin of that idea that had entered into his thinking. Trying to improve his mood, I suggested that we go to the fitness center. We did, but once there, neither fitness center

technicians nor I could convince him of the correct way to con-
vert his pulse rate. Finally we all gave up and a technician recorded it for him.

At home I went about my chores until it occurred to me that
it had been a while since I had heard Job. I found him in our
bedroom sitting in his recliner with his head bowed down almost
to the floor.

"Now, what's wrong," I asked him.

"I don't want to live anymore if you don't want me around,"
was his answer.

"Job, I don't know what you're talking about," I told him.

I wanted to call someone, anyone, A doctor, but which one,
our family doctor or the neurologist? I called Amy at work but
she was away from her desk. Not knowing how Carol felt after
having just giving birth, I felt I could not call her.

Somehow, I got through the evening, but I did not relax.
What new thing is this to add to the pile of stress that already
nests on my heart?

March 7, 2001 (Wednesday)

The sun is out today. Daffodils are way above ground. Some
tree buds are swelling and turning red. Weeping willows are turning green. When I went to Wrightstown I invited Job to ride
along with me. He is in a better mood today and remembers
nothing of yesterday.

March 8, 2001 (Thursday)

The weather is quite moderate on this another sunny day. We
went to the fitness center much later than we usually do. Job had
no trouble at all with the heart rate conversion table. In the afternoon he became restless and went for a walk. When I saw him
turn onto a street where I could no longer see him, I got in the
car and followed him.

March 9, 2001 (Friday)

Job needed to get out for a while, so we went to lunch at a
restaurant that we dine at frequently. I don't care for the food anymore but it is reasonably priced and the restaurant is fairly close
by. While we were there a young man came to our table to speak

to Job. They had worked at the bank together. Job has been retired only twelve years, and under normal circumstances I'm sure the recognition would have been mutual, but Job did not recognize the former coworker. I was glad that the young man made himself known. I know that Job was glad to be recognized and spoken to.

March 12, 2001 (Monday)
We had an appointment with the neurologist today. I was disappointed that Job remembered two words less (fourteen— down from sixteen) on this visit than on the last one. The neurologist has prescribed a different medication that he thinks is a little better than the one currently being used. He has started him on the lowest dosage and will increase the dosage until it reaches the highest level that can be prescribed. He hopes that Job will tolerate the new medication well enough to continue taking it.

March 13, 2001 (Tuesday)
I was awake in time to get to the fitness center by 7:00, the time we usually arrive, but Job was sleeping so peacefully, I wouldn't wake him. We went later, and from there to the mall. I bought three pairs of Calvin Klein pajama bottoms from Bloomingdale's for him. I didn't buy the tops, which is a good thing. The bottoms alone cost ninety-three dollars. I came to my senses after we got home and decided that I will return them tomorrow and look for cheaper ones in Wal-Mart.

March 16, 2001 (Friday)
Happy birthday, Wilma. Today you would be seventy-six. Lois and I remembered.
Job and I went to the city to hear the Philadelphia Orchestra matinee concert. We walked from Market East to the concert hall. The weather was warm and we did not mind the walk, even though it was raining a little. We enjoyed the concert.

March 17, 2001 (Saturday)
Job really needs help with just about everything at the fitness center. Not with the equipment that he does, but with recording things on his chart, and in knowing which piece of equipment to

exercise on next. Today he ignored all the help that I offered, so eventually I didn't offer any. At home he tried to settle into a sulky depression, but I ignored him and the behavior disappeared.

Except for a trip to the library and to K-Mart, we've been in all day. It's moving towards evening now. We've had dinner. I've talked to Carol. Amy has been with her since the baby came. Amy has left for home and Carol misses her. Julian went with Aaron to take Amy to the airport.

March 18, 2001 (Sunday)

After church we packed our bags for going out to see the new baby. I laid out all of Job's things on the bed so that he could pack them himself. Letting him do it this way has worked out much better. After his bags were packed I told him it would be just fine to take them into the living room to wait until we needed them in the morning. He did that, but all afternoon and into the evening he walked back and forth from bedroom to living room fiddling with the bags. Late into the night I finally insisted that he come to bed, or at least stop the pacing as it was making me very nervous. At that, of course, he grew sullen.

March 19, 2001 (Monday)

Our flight to Cincinnati was without turbulence. We took a taxi from the airport so that Carol would not have to bring the two children out. Traveling with Job is difficult. I must keep my eyes on him every minute. He thinks he can wander to the men's room alone, but I know that to let him out of my sight is risky and unwise. I have witnessed him taking off and going the wrong way when he comes out of the men's room. Oh, well.

It was fun trying to figure out whom the baby favors. She kind of favors my mother, but I see traces of Aaron's mother as well. One thing we all agree on, she is a very pretty baby girl.

March 21, 2001 (Tuesday)

We are at Carol's. I was up by 8:00, but Job slept on until 10:00. He tends to understandably get disoriented here in this unfamiliar place. After he got up and was dressed he had a serious bout of something. Confusion? A seizure? He lay supine on the floor, eyes closed, not speaking. I kept talking to him. Our two-year-old grandson Julian brought him orange juice. Whatever frightening thing it was that happened didn't last long. Was it the orange juice that helped? When he was okay we walked to the supermarket. Since we are missing our exercise regimen I thought the walk would be good for him.

March 23, 2001 (Friday)

Job is no less confused here than he is at home. He doesn't seem any happier here than at home either. Julian loves him so much and wants him to play with him, but he doesn't. How I wish Julian could have known him before this mental decline. They both would have enjoyed each other.

March 24, 2001 (Saturday)

It's Job's birthday. We gave him cards. Carol bought a cake and we sang "Happy Birthday." Julian joined in the singing. Job remembered the month and date of his birth, but he couldn't remember the year. We tried to play a game of dominoes but he got darkly confused and we had to stop.

March 25, 2001 (Sunday)

Alana was baptized today. She wore the same dress that her mother and aunt wore for their baptisms. Carol had the christening today so that we could be here for it.

March 28, 2001 (Wednesday)

In two more days we will go home. Job and I, and I suspect Aaron and Carol as well are ready for that to happen. With two babies, I thought Carol would need my help for two weeks otherwise I would not have committed to such a long stay. It is hard on all of us. Her routine is upset as is ours. Our extended stay has given her a chance to see some of the difficulties I am having with her father.

March 31, 2001 (Saturday)

I did the packing for both of us. Early in the morning the bags were packed and setting by the doorway. Carol, Job, Julian and I decided to go to lunch. With Julian in his stroller, we walked down to Hyde Park Square. We ate in a little restaurant called "Indigo." When we returned from the Square it was time to head for the airport. Aaron and Julian drove us there. Julian was asleep by the time we arrived at the airport.

We had a good flight home and made good connections with the train that would take us to our little town. At home, Job went right to bed. I put away our clothes and got his medicines for the week together before I went.

TWENTY-THREE

April 1, 2001 (Sunday)

I am glad to be home but I feel real teary. I guess it's the let-down from being around lively little Julian. Carol is also good with her father. Since she is not around him all the time, so she has more patience to let him help her do things. It doesn't tire her out repeating every direction many times. I also feel very alone.

Job has had several attacks of shortness of breath. He doesn't appear to be sick, and when I ask him if he is he says, no, that he's okay.

We went to church. The day is overcast, with rain in the forecast. It is the first day of daylight saving time, and the day has seemed long. All day I've heard an owl crying it's mournful thoughts. I've noticed that they begin talking by early February. It always sounds as if there is only one of them.

There are lots of cars near Berman's house. I wonder if he is sick or just has a lot of company. We almost never have company. When the children come for visits, our house comes alive. It becomes once more, a home, with life, and breath, and happiness.

April 5, 2001 (Thursday)

I acted as surrogate grandmother to a little four-year-old red-head at the annual Grandmothers' Tea Party. I guess his real grandmother lives too far away to attend. Today has been like spring, warm.

April 6, 2001 (Friday)

It is a dreary, dreary day. I've tried with minimal success to be rid of a quasi-sinus headache. Job has been quiet all day and has hardly spoken a word to me. I presume he is sulking about something but I have been too sick to care or ponder the cause. Why hasn't Lois called?

April 9, 2001 (Monday)

It is warm enough that I hung part of my wash outside. I understand that there are communities where that is not ALLOWED. My, my, how hoity toidy we have grown as a society. What harm could it do to property values to hang your wash on a line outside? I hope I never become affluent enough to be able to afford to live among such snobbery.

A social worker from the County Agency on Aging visited us today. I thought we might be entitled to financial aid for Job, but we don't qualify. The social worker said we are considered "middle income." I guess we are—right in the middle of needing more income.

For our outing we went to Burpee's. Job bought tomato seeds, which he brought home and didn't bother to plant.

As dusk came, I sat on our back steps and listened to birds sing. If you listen very carefully you can distinguish between when they are singing and when they are talking.

April 10, 2001 (Tuesday)

Job has been good all day. I shudder to think what tomorrow will bring. It is night now, the time when I feel most useless. I have time to think, and my thoughts are mostly, 'why am I here on planet Earth.'

April 11, 2001 (Wednesday)

Already it is 8:00 at night. The day seems to have gone before it began. I went to prepare breakfast. When I returned to the bedroom Job was coming out of the bathroom holding the jacket to his good, gray suit in his hand. As gently as I could, I told him—again—that it was not Sunday and we were not going anywhere where he needed to be dressed up. He said he didn't know what he was doing.

Only gloomy blackness describes his mood. I had to ask him repeatedly to take off the trousers to the suit and hang them in the closet. So, you see, the day began badly for me. I was committed to going to Wrightstown, but I didn't want to leave him alone. His mood brightened a fraction and I did go but was anxious the three hours that I was away and he was alone.

We went to the supermarket when I got home. I got dinner together and put the garbage out. I am starting to feel useless. I don't like mingling with people. In the mostly white world that we live in, my skin seems dark, "well nigh to blackness," and my eyes have no sparkle.

April 12, 2001 (Thursday)

There was a church service tonight commemorating Maundy Thursday. I made no effort to attend it. Job would have been the one wanting to attend and he hasn't a notion of what day it is. He has been a bit mentally fuzzy today. During the day we had our differences, but things were better by nightfall. We watched TV together. I was in bed first. When I saw him searching for his pajamas I got up and helped him find them. When he got into bed he moved very close to me—old time close—and without saying a word, put his arms around me, and laid his head on my shoulder. I can't remember the last time that happened. He seems so tired, so awfully, awfully tired.

April 14, 2001 (Saturday)

Amy and James are visiting for the weekend. I am so proud of her for coming up as often as she can to help with her father. I wanted to go to the city to give Lois a hand but was forbidden to do so. Amy wanted me to have the day to myself to do whatever I wanted to do. She thought I would go out somewhere. I meant to but got busy catching up on things I never have time to do when I have no one to help me.

I know that Carol would come also, but she lives too far away. Amy prepared breakfast. Then she and her father went out. They were out for most of the morning and afternoon. When they came home at five o'clock, she apologized for not having kept him out longer.

Being at home alone for a short time was very pleasant, but I knew that Job would be coming home. I still cannot imagine what life would be like if it were a certainty that he would never come home again.

April 15, 2001 (Easter Sunday)

We went to church, which as usual on Easter Sunday was filled to capacity. I was glad that I had prepared most of my dinner for today yesterday. Otherwise I would have been quite frazzled trying to get it together.

It was almost 6:00 when Amy left for home. Afterwards I walked in our backyard near a flowerbed with a patch of daffodils. A pale yellow butterfly flew close to me.

Amy has called to say that she and James arrived home safely. Job is in bed. The house is quiet. I am alone again.

April 16, 2001 (Monday)

It is night again, almost 10:30, but what a day it has been. Actually, I should start with last night. Job had gone to bed early and by 11:30 was up again, insisting that he had to get up and go to work.

"But you are retired," I told him. He was not convinced and gave me a very hard time. It was disconcerting.

This morning he seemed better. He came out to breakfast in the kind of casual clothes I would expect him to wear on a day when nothing was planned. I had to remind him—insist upon it— to brush his teeth. Many mornings I think he doesn't brush them. When breakfast was over he went into the bedroom and put on a tie with the any-old-kind-of shirt he was wearing. With that he put on the jacket to his best gray suit and laid his gray felt hat on the chair. The way he wears the hat, with the brim turned down all the way around, reminds me of characters in gangster movies. We were only going to the city to visit my sister, and he has a more casual hat that he could have worn, but I didn't even suggest that he change his outfit.

During the day he finally settled down to a normal, uneasy, restlessness.

Grass is getting green. Leaves are forming on trees. Our forsythia bushes are blooming, as are daffodils and hyacinths. My world is quiet and sad. I called Carol but she was busy and said she would call back. She didn't. It's okay. She has her hands full taking care of two babies.

April 18, 2001 (Wednesday)

This year seems so different from all others that I can remember. Days seem short because they are all filled up with my doing things. I must do everything that needs to be done both inside and outside of the house. I now prepare Job's breakfast.

April 19, 2001 (Thursday)

Job had his four-month physical examination today. His physical health is good. Our doctor was in a very conversational mood today. The subject of belief in God came up. The doctor said he believes in God but isn't sure about other religious complexities. I remarked that if I were not a Christian I would incline toward Buddhism, although I have no interest in being reincarnated. But if I were reincarnated I would want my new life to be that of a leaf, or flower, or something that helps nature reproduce itself.

Dr. Miles has treated our illnesses for years. When I am in for my examinations he often remarks about the pity of Job's dementia, noting his mother had also been a victim of the disease.

"Here's a man," he would say, "who would come into my office with big books, and they were not for show. He had actually read them."

The doctor was absolutely right.

April 20, 2001 (Thursday)

It is getting very warm, so I took down the storm windows and put the window screens in today. It is a job, of course, that Job has always done and could have helped with, but he made no effort to do so.

He has been all turned around today. Up and dressed by 7:30, he announced that he was going for a walk down the street. I don't like for him to go alone for walks but today I was too tired to worry about it. Fortunately, he came back.

When I went for my appointment with the ophthalmologist I left him sitting in the living room reading the newspaper. That's where he was when I returned home. We usually have dinner at 5:00. At 4:00 he went to the kitchen and ate cereal and other breakfast items. At 5:00 I called him to dinner and he ate. With that over he put on his jacket and hat and asked if that was "all right to wear."

"To wear where? I asked.

"I don't know. Where are we going tonight?" He wanted to know.

I never know where his mind is, where his thoughts are.

[I do not know at this point that this behavior will become more habitual and more troublesome as time goes by. Right now, my concern is what will he do when night comes.]

April 22, 2001 (Sunday)

After we came from church, Job sat in the bedroom sleeping. He slept for several hours. Eventually he went into the kitchen and ate a bowl of cereal. I had set the table, as we would shortly eat dinner. We ate. Not much conversation passed between us. What little did, I initiated. I initiate most of our conversations.

By 7:00, he was in bed, but he got up several hours later and washed himself in the bathroom sink and was about to get dressed when I told him he needed to stay in bed. He did, with much coaxing, return to bed only to get up again an hour or so later and repeat the process. This time I got out of bed and removed the keys used to lock the doors with deadbolts. A key has always been left in front and back doors. He was very, very restless and uncommunicative. This time I did not try to coax him back to bed, although he did return after a long time of sitting up. Not until then did I fall asleep.

TWENTY-FOUR

❦

April 23, 2001 (Monday)

Oh God, Oh God! What is happening? This has been Job's worst day yet. It started out okay. He went outside to bring in the newspaper. I was in the bedroom, so some time passed before I came to the front of our ranch house. It might have been the unusual quietness that prompted me to go there. I don't know.

What I do know is that Job was nowhere to be found, not in the living room, nor in the yard. Nor did I sight him when I looked up and down our street. I panicked. I threw a robe over nightclothes, jumped into the car and went looking for him. When I didn't see him I called 911 because I was too nervous to find the number of the local police.

I was in tears, not knowing what to do. I called our daughter Carol in Ohio. While I was on the telephone with her, he came in. I just didn't want to talk to him. I gave him the phone and he talked to Carol. She must have asked him where he had been.

"I went for a long walk," I heard him tell her. She must have asked him where he went.

"I walked all the way up to the top of the hill," he said.

'What hill, I thought to myself. Was it the hill on our street?' I wondered. Then why didn't I see him when I went in the car to look for him?'

All day he has acted positively crazy. He paces back and forth, from the front of the house to the back of it. He sits down and jumps right back up. He says almost nothing, and what he does say makes no sense.

Can it be that the new medication is having a reverse affect

than intended and is making his condition worse instead of better? The neurologist had said (I thought) that this medication
would not only slow the progression of Alzheimer's, but might
possibly reverse the dementia. I must have misunderstood him.

Trash pickup day in our development is Monday, so it is put
to curbside on Sunday night. By accident I noticed that recepta-
cles of our neighbors were still out, while ours was not. I knew
I had set it out last night. I checked in the back and discovered
that the receptacle was there and had been emptied. Inside of it
a large, brown paper bag such as is used to line kitchen waste-
baskets had been placed.

Where was the garbage? I found it dumped onto the compost
pile. We do compost, but included in what was dumped was
garbage that should not have been put there. I had to pick the
garbage up, put it back into the can and put it back out to the
curb for collection.

The events of today are too numerous to set down in writing. Job would sit down and hop up again almost before his bottom made contact with the chair. Clearly, he was agitated but in
a way that I had never witnessed before.

If I asked him a question his answer was never related to the
question. Also, in whatever response he made he would add
additional unrelated information.

At one point I became so exasperated I yelled, "Job, you simply must sit down. I am too tired to keep following after you,
and you're driving me crazy!"

He went to bed fairly early and slept through the night. I was
afraid anticipating how he would be when he woke up. I didn't
know but what he would be a completely babbling, totally demen-
ted person. As usual, I prayed before going to bed. I was too weary
to ask any petition of God except that He let His will be done.
And yet, perhaps tiredness had nothing to do with my prayer.
Maybe I have just resigned myself to the understanding that God's
Will is being done and there is nothing I can do about it.

April 24, 2001 (Tuesday)

He is better today, thank God, but I know that it is a tenu-
ous repose. Throughout the day he still said irrational things, but
by and large he has been himself. He watched "Matlock" on the

TV. However, off and on, he dozed.

Yesterday he had begun mowing the lawn but stopped when the mower became wedged between two trees and Job left it there. I had to go to Wrightown. Before leaving I made him promise not to try to get the lawnmower unstuck, and not to try to mow the lawn. When I got home the lawnmower had been unstuck, and some grass had been cut. He doesn't remember how he got the mower from between the trees. He has no memory of cutting the grass.

April 25, 2001 (Wednesday)

Today is Amy and James' third Anniversary. We are watching the nightly news. Where did the day go? Granted, I slept—or stayed in bed—a bit longer than usual. I encouraged Job to do the same.

He has been frighteningly good today. He sat in the living room reading the paper for a long time, just as he used to do. He has talked to me more than he has for a long, long time, even being snippy on one occasion. I'm still keyed up remembering Monday's episode. I keep wondering what tomorrow, or indeed what the next minute will bring in Job's behavior.

The Reverend Leon Sullivan died today of leukemia.

The weather has cooled down a great deal from what it has been for the past two days. I had to put the heat up a little. Job even needed the portable heater in our bedroom on.

April 26, 2001 (Thursday)

I thought it best not to leave Job at home alone, so he went with me to Wrightstown. In the afternoon we had an interview with the coordinator of an adult day care center. Our doctor has suggested that I leave Job in one for three days a week so that I can have some free time, but I've been reluctant to even consider it. Now, I am feeling, as well as seeing, the need to do so.

The interview was long and tiring. Most of the clients have some form of dementia, some cases are worse than are others. A few are left at Elder Care simply because no one is at home to care for them.

I hate the thought of leaving Job in the same environment with the worst cases that I saw. Still, to know that he is secure in that setting is preferable to leaving him alone. The program seems to offer activities that may prove beneficial to him. If nothing else, it will be a good social outlet for him. I wish there were someone living in my household that I could confer with to help me make decisions.

April 27, 2001 (Friday)

We went to the Academy of Music for our matinee concert. Today's program was music by Smetana. Maestro Sawalich conducted. The orchestra played so movingly, Job wept. I love "The Moldou" and felt like weeping also. I had thought we would have dinner while downtown, but we came back to our area and ate.

April 30, 2001 (Monday)

Job has acted peculiarly today. I wanted time to myself, so in the early morning, while he slept, I crept into the kitchen and ate grapefruit and enjoyed a leisurely cup of coffee. I finished the "jumble" and "cryptogram" in the paper, then prepared his breakfast.

He slept until 9:00. I found him in the bedroom with a clean T-shirt on but he had not taken off his pajama bottoms and was confused about what to do next. Very gently I reminded him several times that what he needed to do next was remove the bottoms and put on a pair of shorts. When he still did not understand, I got the shorts from the drawer for him and left him to finish dressing.

He has been quiet, quiet, quiet all day. He sat in a chair in the living room and appeared to be sleeping. He went into the kitchen and set the table for dinner. We ate. He washed the dishes, then it was back to the bedroom, where he sat in his recliner and slept.

It is 8:00 and he is in bed. I've put the deadbolts on and removed the keys from the doors, as he is sure to get up an hour from now and dress for going out.

Today was my free day, but his behavior upset me so, I didn't do anything pleasant with it.

May 1, 2001 (Tuesday)

For a while I thought he wasn't going to the fitness center, he slept so late. I didn't push it. I knew that I would not go without him. When he finally came out of the bedroom he was dressed for going to church, or some place where dressing up was required.

I didn't challenge his wearing a dress suit, but I suggested that he might want to take the tie off, since he would wear sneakers instead of dress shoes. Surprisingly, he was cooperative. In the afternoon Carol called and talked with him. She wanted to know how he felt, and he told her that he felt fine.

He is in his quiet mode today. It is not as acute as it was yesterday. We stopped at Boston Market and bought lemonade and sat in the restaurant to drink it. We went to Burpee seed store and bought tomato plants. That will give him something to work on tomorrow—if he will do it.

I had a letter from my friend whose husband has for years suffered from a different kind of dementia from Job's. Her letter was in response to one I had written to her.

"Dear Lori," I had written, "sometimes things get so bad, I want to go somewhere where no one can hear me and scream, and scream, and scream!" In her reply she said that she just goes into another room and cries. I always want to cry but the tears never come.

It is 8:20. Job is undressed for bed.

May 2, 2001 (Wednesday)

Today is Angie's (my brother) birthday. He is eighty-one but doesn't look it. He is very fit, and his mind is sharp.

Dinner was simple. I made an omelette. Our green vegetable was a tossed salad. I had put a bottle of hot sauce on the table in case Job wanted a bit on his omelette. When I wasn't looking I think he put hot sauce on his salad as if it were salad dressing, and when he tasted the salad he complained that it was too hot. He left his dinner on the table and didn't return to it. I cleaned up the kitchen.

We both went to bed at approximately the same time, but he was very restless and didn't fall asleep. He was restless and tossed and turned almost frantically. His continuous movement kept me awake, and I finally got up and sat in his recliner until he fell asleep, which seemed like hours later.

Amy had called earlier to tell me that she had found a lump in her breast that has been diagnosed as benign. She told me not to worry. Sure. And tell the water that tumbles over Niagra Falls to stop falling.

May 3, 2001 (Thursday)

We went to the fitness center early. Job was thoroughly con-fused. Is the new medicine really better than the one he has been taking? It doesn't seem so. What do I do? I've called the neurol-ogist.

Late this afternoon Amy called. Like me, she doesn't want daddy in Elder Care with clients who appear older and "more out of it" than he seems to be. He has been quiet all day but seems better this early evening. We sat in the front yard togeth-er for a while.

May 4, 2001 (Friday)

The weather is very hot for this early part of May. The tem-perature went up to the nineties. Job mowed about half of the lawn and stopped. I had a feeling that once he stopped he would not finish, but he said he had only stopped to rest. We do have a large area to cut. He did go back to the job and finished mow-ing all but a spot about ten tractor turns in size. When I asked if he would finish that tiny spot tomorrow he said, "maybe."

We went to see a movie and to dinner afterwards. Job said he would shower and shave before we went, but he didn't.

Daffodils have ended their short life. Tulips have lost their stately posture. The petals have opened wide, indicating that they too will soon disappear. Lilacs have had their bright moment of the season and are fading, as all life does. Only the azalea bush on the north side of the house is still enjoying life. It was crowd-ed in the space where it was originally. In its present location it has spread to take up most of the side of the house.

May 5, 2001 (Saturday)

I knew he would not cut that tiny patch of lawn. I asked him to and he did as he does when he is angry. He huffed up, start-ed the lawnmower and set about covering the same ground that was mowed yesterday. Over and over again the lawnmower went covering the same ground it covered yesterday. I went out and showed him the little patch that needed cutting. He simply ignored me. Finally I got out the reel mower and cut the little patch myself. After I did that and had gone back inside, he went over the spot with the tractor mower.

May 6, 2001 (Sunday)

Not that it did any good, but I let Job know how angry I was about the lawn incident yesterday.

May 7, 2001 (Monday)

Our yard is so beautiful. The grass is like green velvet. Flowers are in bloom all over it. I spent the morning trimming overgrown spirea bushes. What a job that was, but I thought it should be done to keep Job from being snatched from the lawn-mower by a branch.

I went for a short visit to my friend Marty. She wasn't in, so I came home. It is a good thing I did. Job was mowing the lawn again after just having mowed it on Saturday. He just does not know what he is doing. Tonight several doctors discussed the disease on TV. Alzheimer's is the cause of death for those afflicted by it. Listening to the discussion I felt drained. Down. I must watch Job's brain shut down, watch it refuse to direct him in executing the simplest tasks.

May 8, 2001 (Tuesday)

ElderMed sponsored a tea and I had planned to attend. It was to be a really fancy affair, so I had bought a hat to wear to it. When last week Job was so bad mentally I decided that I could not leave him alone to attend the tea. The hat is in Amy's old room. I probably will never wear it.

May 9, 2001 (Wednesday)

It must be the new medication that is affecting Job's mood and behavior. Today has been bad, bad, bad. Last night was also, in a way. He went to bed looking for his condoms. I noticed him on occasion opening and closing his dresser drawers. He would open a drawer, search through underwear, then close them it. He repeated the action over and over again, searching each of the four drawers. When I asked what he was looking for he said he was looking for his condoms.

Condoms were not the method of birth control that we had used, so I was not familiar with them. I had in mind that to use them would require an erect penis, and since his prostate opera-tion ten years earlier, Job hadn't had one.

At first it was really funny.

"Why do you need condoms," I asked.

"So you won't get pregnant," he answered, with all of the seriousness of a newly married groom to his bride.

I told him it was not likely that I would become pregnant since I was almost seventy-three-years old.

This morning, he doesn't even remember that we are married.

"Why are you here?" he asked me.

"Why am I here?" I said. "I belong here."

"You do," he said pleasantly enough, "why?"

"Because I live here. I'm your wife."

When he asked if we had children I became really alarmed. I took him into the living room and showed him high school graduation pictures of our girls that were sitting in frames on the piano. He knew their names but I am not sure if he knew they were his children. His mood was good. I didn't convince him that I was his wife, but at several different times throughout the day he said that I seemed to be a nice person, and he would be will-ing to marry me. I screamed. I cried. I said, Job please do not ask me that (if we were married) again.

I thought it best not to tell our children about this episode.

* * *

WE BOTH GET PHYSICAL CHECKUPS twice a year. On one of the six-month visits I would be given a breast examination and PAP smear, as well as being examined for other conditions that might affect my health. On one of Job's six-month visits, he would be given a digital rectal examination.

I remember well the visit on which the doctor discovered an irregularity on Job's prostate and referred him to an urologist to have it checked. The urologist performed a needle biopsy and confirmed that the prostate should be treated. For a person of Job's age, sixty-four at the time, he suggested surgery rather than radiation or other form of treatment.

We prepared for the surgery knowing that it might result in Job's becoming impotent. The urologist/surgeon assured us that he would do all that he could to prevent this from happening.

The night before his hospitalization I wept at the thought of what could happen. Job was very reassuring that everything would be all right, but it has never been "all right" again. After the surgery, Job could have gotten injections that would have effected an erection, but he would have had to go to the doctor's office to get them. Also, this would have destroyed any possibility of the lovemaking act being spontaneous so neither of us found this acceptable. We also spurned other gadgets on the market that might have worked. I simply was unwilling to subject Job to experimenting with them. The operation has not diminished our love for each other, it has merely curtailed our capacity to fully express it.

* * *

May 10, 2001 (Thursday)

He is being very contrary today. I can always differentiate when he is doing what he has always done and what he does because of Alzheimer's. He knows that he has done something to make me angry, so he is going out of his way to generate conversation, something that lately he never does.

May 12, 2001 (Saturday)

We are at Amy's. She insists that I stay home and rest. She and daddy went to the nursery for plants. She wants Job to help her select some, and also help her set them out. It will give him something to do. While they were out I read and solved cryptogram puzzles.

May 14, 2001 (Monday)

We're home again, and the lump in my throat is back. I simply am tired of dealing with Job alone. In any situation it is so difficult knowing what to do or say to him.

While we were away the handyman I engaged to prepare our vegetable garden plot did so. At first Job said he would work in the garden, but he insisted on plowing it first with his own rotor tiller. I told him patiently and repeatedly that the ground was already prepared for planting. He went right ahead with what he was doing as if he were on one planet and I on another where communicating with each other was not possible. Oh, God! What can I do?

TWENTY-FIVE

❦

May 18, 2001 (Friday)

Yesterday I had my colonoscopy. After I got home I slept for most of the afternoon. I had engaged a nurse to stay with Job while I went for my procedure. This morning he was extremely confused. He didn't eat all of his breakfast neither did he eat all of his dinner. Maybe it is not because he is losing his appetite but because of lack of variety in the way meals are prepared. In the morning I am going to prepare something different for him.

We have watched the 11:00 news and are headed for bed. I dread going because there's always the sex thing. I've always tried to be sensitive to his physical needs and respond to them, but somehow this seems different, more like a lecherous obsession, and I am repulsed by it. I've concluded that it has something to do with the new medication for Alzheimer's that he has been taking since April.

I need emotional help, but where can I get it? Who is the right person to talk to? A doctor perhaps? That would be so embarrassing. I've never had a confidant.

Amy had surgery to have the lump in her breast removed. She called and said that she is all right.

May 19, 2001 (Saturday)

We went to the fitness center and Michael saw to it that Job did all of the pieces of equipment that he is scheduled for. Michael is a very nice young man.

The morning was gray but in the afternoon the sun came out. Job pulled up a few weeds and said he should mow the lawn but made no effort to do so.

We had a simple dinner of tacos (ground turkey filling), French fries, and applesauce. Job said repeatedly that it was good, still, he picked at it as if he didn't care for it.

We watched the evening news. Afterwards, he grew silent and put on his long, doleful face. He talked at length about how he could not have intercourse (because of his impotence after prostate surgery), and did I think he was "queer," or think less of him for that. I could neither reassure him nor divert his attention to another topic.

At 9:00 we went to the rec. room to watch a TV "Colombo" movie. He excused himself from watching and came upstairs, but said he would be "right back." I suspected the reason for his mission and went to check on him. When I asked him what he was searching for among his underwear in his dresser drawer, he said he was looking to see if he had any condoms.

When we got into bed I was adamant that he wasn't to bother me so he might as well keep his pajama bottoms on and button up the shirt top.

May 20, 2001 (Sunday)

Today was bad, bad, bad, although it started out well enough. He showered willingly and didn't resist brushing his teeth when I reminded him that he had forgotten to do so. I went to the kitchen to prepare breakfast, and when he came out of the bedroom he was breathing rapidly and heavily (until the cardiologist told me there was a difference, I described it as hyperventilating). And his mood, dark and brooding, was like midnight in a thick, thick forest.

He would not lift up his head. It was as if a heavy yoke placed around his neck kept him from doing so. He ate only a scant portion of his breakfast. At church he refused to take Communion. When I asked him why he said he didn't know why.

I called Carol to tell her that his condition is worsening. She took the report well, and said she knew. She and Amy do know what they get from the Internet, which they visit often to get information on the disease. But they do not really know. Their thinking that they REALLY have more than an academic understanding of what is going on with their father is like a man's understanding of what childbirth is like.

I made tuna sandwiches for lunch. I cut a piece of cake for both of us. I left his lunch on the table and went from the room. I simply cannot stand to witness that dark, dark downward looking countenance, and hear that heavy, almost sensual, breathing.

May 21, 2001 (Monday)
Blue, blue Monday. May is slipping away. Job is slipping away into a world away from my world into one of his own. I see him trying, but he simply can not force himself to eat. I FRIED chicken, made gravy, cooked spinach, and rice, all dishes that any African/American would delight in eating, but after only a few forkfuls, Job left the rest uneaten.

Towards evening he perked up a bit and was able to tell me that when he tries to eat he gets a queasy feeling in his stomach. I've made an appointment with our doctor for Thursday. I hate to wait until then, but I am grateful that he can see us as soon as that.

May 22, 2001 (Tuesday)
He still cannot eat, and he has noticeably lost weight. He must be the only person in the whole world who certainly does not need to lose weight.

He went to the back of our yard just to look around. When he came in he was reeling, as if he might fall down. He said he was out of breath. He managed to get to the bedroom, where he fell across the bed and slept for most of the afternoon. For lunch I gave him chicken broth, and for dinner, soup.

Without asking the advice of the doctor, at bedtime I didn't give him the new medication that he has been taking for Alzheimer's.

May 23, 2001 (Wednesday)
I had called the neurologist. Today he returned my call. He says it sounds like the new medication is not agreeing with Job. I'm to continue giving him one 4.5mg pill instead of two a day for the rest of the week, then stop it altogether. We have an appointment to see the neurologist on June seventh.

May 24, 2001 (Thursday)
We kept our appointment with Dr. Miles. He filled out the

necessary forms for me to take Job to Elder Care. He advised me not to feel guilty about doing so.

From the doctor's office we went to the closing day picnic of the Wrightstown Friends Nursery School.

Amy is home. She came up for the thirtieth Anniversary celebration of Madrigals, the music group she sang with in High School. Afterwards we went to "Friday's" for snacks.

As we were preparing for bed Job began his nightly ritual of searching for his condoms.

May 25, 2001 (Friday)

We went to Wrightstown Friends (Morning) Nursery School picnic. Already, Job's appetite for eating has improved! However, he is still obsessed with sex.

May 27, 2001 (Sunday)

Amy went to church with Job. She wanted me to stay at home and rest. I appreciate the offer. I didn't get much rest. I cooked dinner so that Amy could eat before starting home. She wanted to leave by two thirty. Job's eating is markedly improved. His obsession with sex is holding steady.

May 28, 2001 (Monday–Memorial Day)

My plan was to visit the cemetery and take flowers for the graves of our loved ones. Our peonies are beautiful. Some flags are open. Together they would have made a beautiful bouquet. I asked Job if he wanted to go. He showed no interest, so I got busy doing other things. Later I was too tired to drive to Rolling Green and reasoned that my loved ones would understand.

Early in the day we went to Burpee's and bought more tomato plants and two pepper plants. We set the plants out and planted two rows of beans.

Job ate all of his dinner and said it was good. The sun has been out all day. The temperature has been comfortable.

May 30, 2001 (Wednesday)

Job didn't start acting peculiar until it was time to go to bed. We had watched an episode of "Matlock." He didn't start wandering about looking for condoms until the show was over. I had hoped that I would be able to tell the neurologist when we meet with him on the seventh that the sex thing was behind us.

He has done a bit of work today—tied down the daffodil stems. I thought that since he was no longer taking the offending medication that he was returning to his old self. I guess that was just wishful thinking.

May 31, 2001 (Thursday)

The month seems to have just begun, and already it is over. Our yard is beautiful with peonies and flags in full bloom.

Minus the medicine that disagreed with him, Job is doing well. He seems more lucid, less depressed, and for the most part is eating normally.

On this last day of May the weather has been beautiful. It has been a bit chilly, but when the sun comes from behind the clouds it is much better.

June 1, 2001 (Friday)

It is almost 11:00 at night. Job has been in bed for about an hour. I think he is asleep and hope that he sleeps through the night. He makes a real production out of preparing for bed. He goes into the bathroom to get undressed, takes out and puts underwear back into dresser drawers many times, folds pants and shirt and leaves them on the chair with several pairs of socks, and engages in sundry idiosyncrasies peculiar to his illness.

He didn't finish all of his dinner, although he said it was good. Later, we ate ice cream.

He didn't do any work, but he did walk in the yard for a while. Yesterday he cultivated the garden.

June 2, 2001 (Saturday)

Exercising at the fitness center for Job began after his heart surgery (1980). I began accompanying him after my bout with sarcoidosis, which required that I take medicine that might cause me to develop osteoporosis. Even though, as mostly everyone says who comes to exercise, I dislike doing the exercises, but I feel better once they are over. Still, if for some reason he doesn't want to go, it provides me with the perfect excuse for not going either. So, on each of the three times a week that we are scheduled to go, I ask him if he feels up to going.

"Are you going to the fitness center today?" I asked him.

"No. I'm too tired," he answered.

"OK. I won't go either," I said, and went into the kitchen and sat down to drink a cup of coffee and do the "jumble" and "cryptogram" puzzles.

When he came into the kitchen dressed for going to workout I was surprised. I dressed hurriedly and we went. He did fine at the fitness center. When we came home he sat and read the newspaper. I decided to work in the yard and he came out and helped. At night he slept well. What a perfectly wonderful day we spent together. The next day—June 3—was also another very good day!

June 4 and June 5, 2001 (Monday and Tuesday)

We went to the travel agency to see about getting plane tickets for our trip to Cincinnati. I stopped at the drugstore to pick up my prescription. We went to Wal-Mart and bought labels for clothing that Job must leave at Elder Care when he goes tomorrow. At night I finished writing ten of nineteen thank you notes that I must write to Morning Friends for the gift they gave me when school closed.

Job continues to look for his condoms and something to do with them once they are found. The very act of his searching repulses me. Oh, cruel, cruel Alzheimer's. Could I in my wildest dreams have considered an overture of affection from Job repulsive? Even now, I do not detest him but the unnaturalness of the action, which I blame firmly and squarely on the new medication.

At Elder Care he didn't hesitate to mingle with other clients. I enjoyed the free time I had without always needing to give him attention, but I did miss him. In the late afternoon we sat outside and enjoyed the flower gardens. Flags are beautiful, as are the peonies, only their fully open petals are already splattering down to the ground.

June 7, 2001 (Thursday)

Our interim appointment with the neurologist was today. They never last long. He has prescribed still another drug for Job's Alzheimer's. I hope it works. I told the doctor that if I noticed any adverse reaction at all I would discontinue the medication and call him right away. I simply can not suffer through another episode of Job's depression and other disturbing behavior. In hindsight, I feel that I waited too long before letting either our primary care doctor or the neurologist know of the deleterious affect the prior drug was having on Job.

While we were out we made a day of it and ate breakfast at IHOP. Since his appetite is still fragile, I ordered from the children's menu for him. That size portion was just enough. He seemed to enjoy it.

June 8, 2001 (Friday)

"What day is it?" he asked.

"Friday," I answered. He went back into the bedroom, and when he came back to the kitchen he was dressed for church.

"Is this all right to wear?" he asked.

"Fine." I answered and continued with my housework. I thought that if he saw that I was not preparing to go out, and since he couldn't drive the car, he would realize that he was overdressed for the day's activities.

When I saw him weeding a flower bed I went out to tell him that I didn't think he wanted to do that work in his nice, light colored suit jacket. I thought he might get grass stain on it.

"And what's wrong with that (wearing the suit jacket)?" he asked.

"Nothing," I answered. "Do whatever your head tells you to do."

He hardly ever says anything to me, often acting as if he is angry. If he is angry, it seems to me, but his memory is such that he doesn't remember things from one second to the next, why does he not forget that he is angry and talk to me?

Actually, I think today he was angry with himself for getting all dressed up on the wrong day for going somewhere special.

It is a beautiful, beautiful day. I love summer. Flowers are all around. Roses are in bloom. Yesterday the lawn was mowed. Our yard is a vision of loveliness.

June 9 through June 13, 2002 (Saturday, Sunday, Monday, Tuesday)

I had a few errands to do this Saturday. Mostly, though, I was relaxed. Toward evening Job began packing for our trip to Ohio.

We won't be leaving until Friday. Nevertheless, he has worked feverishly, stuffing shorts into jacket pockets, piling shirts on top of trousers, and jackets (as many as he can find) on top of jackets. Caps, sneakers, everything. Of course, when I actually pack his bags, all extraneous clothing will be left at home.

I must always check and recheck his bags, for if he sees an extra cap about, he sticks it into one of his bags (or mine). It is maddening. At night I heard him trying the doors—to get out and put his things in the car, I guess. I was glad that I had removed the keys from the locks.

Today (Sunday) has been another perfect one. Job has been very restless today and has kept pacing up and down the hallway, from our bedroom to the living room. He took the first dose of the new medicine this morning, but that has nothing to do with his restlessness.

At night I leave a tiny opening in the draperies. When I peeped through it this Monday morning at around 6:00, through separations in gray/white clouds, I saw a patch of blue sky. I heard Job in the bathroom getting washed in the sink. I was afraid he would get dressed and want to go out, which would mean that I would need to get up as well. I breathed a sigh of relief (and a prayer of thanks) that he merely put on clean underwear and came back to bed, so I slept a while longer.

On this first day of weather with temperatures up to 90 degrees, he came out to breakfast wearing a winter turtleneck sweater. For a while he sat in the living room and read the paper. I had left the door open. He closed it, complaining that he was cold. He went into our bedroom and closed the door and turned on the space heater. There he sat all morning while I went about my work.

I'm worried about him. He does absolutely nothing except wash or dry the dishes. Sometimes I feel guilty that he always does them, so I do them myself. He spends a lot of time sitting with his head down. Last night he had a slight nocturnal bowel accident. Is the new medication causing it?

Early evenings he becomes restless and paces about doing things. Darting here and there, nervously rushing about, opening drawers, stacking his change on top of his dresser, counting the money that's in his wallet over and over, doing any little things that keep him pacing anxiously about.

Tonight it looks as if a storm is coming up. I like to watch storm clouds gather, but I don't like when there's loud thunder and piercing lightning.

Often I walk out to the garden. Our plants need rain.

It is Tuesday and exercise day again. We both went and afterwards I left Job at Elder Care, which is practically next door to the fitness center. He said he didn't mind staying there for a while. I took advantage of my free time by going for the massage that Carol gave me as a Christmas gift.

I picked him up at 3:00. He was fine. I asked him if he would like it if I made an apple pie.

"Well, I like apple pie," he said.

So I rushed and made one, but he didn't eat any of it. He has started that head hung down out-of-breath behavior again. He complains of having a queasy stomach. I guess it's his nerves. It bothers me tremendously. He didn't feel up to helping with the dishes.

In the afternoon he had busied himself with stuffing ties and socks and underwear into pockets of suits. Shirts and sweaters, still on hangers, are bundled together. Belts around the bundles hold the contents together.

On top of the shirt that he had worn all day, he has put on another one. It is almost 8:30 and he has settled into acting more like a normal, non-demented person.

June 14, 2001 (Thursday–Flag Day)

We went by train to Center City to attend Job's annual retirees luncheon. I was afraid Job's memory problem would prevent his recognizing anyone, but there were several former coworkers that he spoke to with apparent full recognition.

The luncheon menu was good. I was glad that he ate all of his food.

It has been very warm today but has cooled some now that it is night. I think I hear crickets singing but surely it is too early in the season for that.

June 25, 2001 (Monday)

We are home from Cincinnati. What a great time we had visiting Carol, Aaron, Julian, and baby Alana. Carol always finds interesting things for us to do. She takes the children for an out-ing every day if only to a park. Job usually went with them. I didn't always, preferring to take advantage of the time to rest and relax.

Job was very cooperative with Carol, and she was very patient with him. I was proud of her for being so. I try always to be patient, and most of the time I succeed. However, for the person who is the constant caregiver, being patient with an Alzheimer's sufferer is sometimes an unaffordable luxury.

Little Julian adores his grandpop. It was at once heartwarm-ing and heartbreaking to see the two of them together. When Job was out of his sight he would always ask, "Where's grandpop?"

"Oh, Carol," I said to Julian's mom, "I wish Julian could have known his grandfather when he wasn't like he is now."

"Well," she said, "he just has to know him as he is."

We had a good flight home and arrived at Philadelphia International Airport by 9:30. We had to go upstairs to collect our luggage, then downstairs again to connect with the regional rail line to bring us to our suburban home.

Our wait for that was almost an hour. The train arrival was on time as scheduled, but it didn't coincide with the arrival time of our flight. Job did not understand this, and during the wait became characteristically restless. Once, when my head was turned for a second or two, he wandered away from where we were sitting. I didn't see him anywhere and was frantic. With my heart racing, I finally spotted him trying to enter a doorway that was clearly marked in large red letters, "DO NOT ENTER." A stairway leading to the upstairs of the airport was beyond the doorway, but we did not need to go upstairs.

"Job, why did you leave where I was sitting?"

"Because I 'm going upstairs."

"We don't need to go back upstairs. We have our luggage, and we must wait here for our train home."

He insisted that he had to go upstairs. I couldn't in any way induce him to sit down. I was both angry and frantic. Who would help me calm him down if he made a scene in this lone-ly place? He stood too close to the yellow marker that designates that you are in danger of being harmed by oncoming trains. His behavior was erratic. He began trying to flag down anything that was moving in any direction—trains, cars, taxicabs, anything moving. I endured almost an hour of this before our train came.

This morning began with another maddening episode of frustration even before we had eaten breakfast. It was during my attempt to prepare breakfast that I discovered that Job's wallet was missing. Needless to say, the discovery was significant enough that everything else was halted and a search for the wallet begun.

Usually, upon retiring to bed, Job would place his wallet either on top of his dresser or in the top drawer of it. When after removing everything from that drawer I didn't find the wallet, I repeated the process, looking through the remaining three drawers without success.

Panic engaged every inch of my being as efforts to locate the wallet proved fruitless. Money wasn't the issue. Very little would have been in the wallet as I had long since stopped allowing him to keep more than fifteen or twenty dollars in it. I did that because he was constantly removing the money and counting it. His bank and social security cards were my concern.

It would be a futile effort I was sure, but one that I must take. I retraced our movements from the night before. We inquired at the train station. Nothing had been turned in there but they suggested that I call the main transportation office. Knowing that it was a useless endeavor, I called. When that source reported that no wallet had been turned in to lost and found, I came home.

In an audacious petition I prayed to God. "Lord, I believe you answer prayers, but I also know that answers do not immediately follow a petition. I don't have time to wait. I need to know if I should start canceling important cards.

Immediately following the prayer I decided to look once more in the drawer where the wallet was usually kept. There, much to my relief, underneath a small sleeve, a cover for an item from his travel kit, was the wallet.

The month of June is moving out. Daylilies are starting to bloom. While we were away hollyhocks grew tall and doubled over from lack of support. Still, they are beautiful. The lawn has been freshly mowed. I've washed the laundry that was brought home dirty.

Dressed in trousers from his good summer suit, white shirt, and tie, Job has done quite a bit of weeding. I am always glad that he shows initiative to do something.

It is evening. I hear children playing. All day it was warm but now it is cool. A bird sings loudly. I feel tired. What is Julian doing? I miss him. He's so much fun.

June 26, 2001 (Tuesday)

Getting back into the routine of going to the fitness center was difficult after such a long time away from it. I left Job at Elder Care for only four hours instead of a full day. When I arrived he was in the hallway talking to a staff member. He was telling her that "his wife" was coming soon to take him home.

His mood was so good I suggested that we go to "Rita's" and get a gelati. He agreed, however when we got home he began to act strange, putting the gelati into the freezer and setting the table for lunch, although he had just eaten before leaving the Center. Instead of milk, he used "Ensure" to mix with something that he didn't eat, and he was just generally sullen and down looking for the rest of the day.

I have no time to sit on the patio and think summer thoughts. We've not even put up a patio umbrella.

June 27, 2001 (Wednesday)

With no fitness center to go to, I consider this a free day. I had done some typing for Marty. She had come early—around nineish—to pick it up. When she left to go home, we went to the train station. We went to Center City to get Job's razor repaired. It didn't need repairing but he complained every time he used it, saying that it didn't work. He had complained about the old one that he had used for many years, so when Carol was home at Christmas time I threw the old one out and she carried him to the store and bought another one. He came home and fished the old one out of the trash and never used the new one.

We found the repair shop without difficulty. After the razor was repaired we had lunch in the food court of the Bellvue, then got the 2:10 train back home. We went directly from the train station to the supermarket and did a modicum of marketing. Immediately when we came home I began getting dinner together.

I was dead tired, but Job had it in his head that we were going someplace. He began packing. He took down all of his shirts from hangers they were on in the closet. Working feverishly, he removed all of his underwear from drawers. Every pair of shoes he owns was removed from the closet, as well as ties and suits. At some point he urged me to pack things up also, as we needed to have everything out of the house by a certain time.

I was too tired to answer or try to stop him. Eventually I asked him to please put things away. Surprisingly, he did, and afterwards acted in a fairly normal way.

The temperature has been in the nineties but there is not much humidity, so the day has been pleasant. Tomorrow promises to be worse. Carol called and I said hello to Julian.

June 30, 2001 (Saturday)

In a few hours June will be history. Today is more humid than yesterday. I bought another small fan for the back of the house and left the air conditioner to cool the front.

June left lilies, daylilies, and black-eyed Susans abloom. Through the little crack in the draperies that I leave open for air to come in at night, I see an occasional firefly flying high up in the trees. There are no crickets yet, just quiet, dark nights.

TWENTY-SIX

I reach for her (his) hand
It's always there.
How long does it last?
Can love be measured by the hours in a day?
I have no answers, but this much I can say:
I know I'll need her (him) 'til the stars all burn away
And she'll (he'll) be there.

IT IS TIME FOR MORE TO BECOME KNOWN ABOUT the Job that exist-ed before plaque invaded his brain and is effecting a complete metamorphosis in the person I have vowed to love, honor, and obey in sickness and in health 'till death do us part.

The mechanics of writing about the bad part is easy. I have only to open composition book after composition book and copy from notes written in black and white on an almost daily basis. The act of telling about the good part is more difficult because my source material, unlike records stored on microfiche, or in the memory bank of a computer, or indeed, written down on paper, is stored only in my mind and heart.

He wanted to be married, he said, and didn't understand my hesitation in accepting his proposal. So I finally told him my rea-son for procrastinating. I didn't want to have a lot of children, wasn't sure in fact if I wanted any at all, but I didn't know how not to have them.

We laughed at the thought of what a shocking revelation that would have been to the little old ladies (and some of my peers) whose eyes, I'm sure, were ever watchful for the telltale disten-tion in my midriff signaling that I was pregnant out of wedlock.

However, journalistic integrity compels me to give credit to Job's principled discipline more than to my steadfast virtue for giving the lie to their suspicions.

Needless to say, Job wasted no time in finding the answer that would solve my dilemma and put an end to his frustration.

We went together to City Hall for our blood test, and to the doctor who had attended him since childhood for our premarital examinations. He saw the doctor first. When I offered the five-dollar fee to the doctor after my examination, he informed me that Job had already paid it. We were on our way to becoming husband and wife.

Our marriage took place on the last Saturday in February, in the year nineteen hundred and fifty seven. The day offered forth a mixture of sunshine, overcast sky, a little shower of rain, and a scant dusting of snow.

"That's how our lives will be," I said to Job, "some days will be sunny, some dreary with unpleasantness, and some will be dark, like an overcast sky." I didn't know how accurate my prophecy would prove to be.

Pastors from both of our churches officiated at the simple wedding ceremony, with my only attendant being one of my six sisters. Job's "Best Man" was one of his two brothers. In an ankle-length, princess style wedding dress and borrowed headpiece, I walked down the aisle of my church on the arm of my father to the altar where a broadly smiling Job awaited.

Postponing a honeymoon until a later date, after the wedding we ate a late supper at our favorite restaurant, then spent our wedding night in the duplex apartment that Job owned and had lived alone on the first floor of it for about a year.

After the first few weeks of being married, I think we both were as blissfully happy as storybooks falsely lead you to believe you will always be. I knew that I was happy, and felt that Job was as well. He certainly seemed to be. One day as I sat by the window watching for him to come home from work, I noticed that as he passed row house after row house and was getting close to apartment, his steps quickened to an almost running pace.

A few months into our marriage Job said there was something he must tell me. It had come to the ears of the pastor of his church that a young woman was claiming that Job was the father of her child, and that "in our quiet moments," Job must tell me about it.

So certain I was of the mendacity of the accusation that had I proper license I could have notarized the falsity of the claim myself. For I felt in possession of a certain sure knowledge that Job was not the father of the unfortunate young woman's child.

However, no action to put the rumor to rest was needed, as it was known generally that the accusing young woman was mentally challenged and had merely manufactured her story.

These forty odd years later, I can say without fear of being in error, that if Job had had any thought, however remote, that he might have been the child's father, he would have insisted on taking responsibility for it in all of the ways that a father should.

Although he wanted a family—children of his own—Job respected my desire to wait before having any. So five years went by before our son, Mark, was born. Before his birth we went on wonderful vacations together, and otherwise went our separate ways, doing things of individual interest. We continued to be active in our respective churches, and I continued to help with caring for my aging parents.

There must have been a reason for my needing to know about family planning before marriage, and I believe the reason was this: Job and I were very compatible and took pleasure in satisfying each other's needs. This made us experience a happiness with each other that seemed selfish not to share with others. Mark's birth was our way of sharing with the world the happiness we felt privately. I also felt it was my duty to God to, as stated in the Old Testament, have children to be raised up to praise Him.

Men do cry. The tragic death of our son three months after his birth caused Job to express his sorrow with weeping, though not in my presence. I heard him sobbing in the bathroom on the morning after the tragedy. For me, he was strong and comforting, with only a subtle external showing of the hurt he felt inwardly. Sudden Infant Death Syndrome was certified as the cause of our baby's death. We'll never know. Our baby was left with a responsible, mature woman sitter while we went to work, and while he was there, he died.

We mourned the death of our son for a long time. Almost

two years later our daughter Carol was born, and two and three-quarter years after that her sister Amy was born. I had returned to work after Mark's death. I did not return to work following the birth of Carol and Amy.

Job was an exemplary father, and continued to be a wonderful husband. He delighted in his children. Carol, of course, was the first benefactor of his affection. In a way, I can detect the great, silent suffering she is enduring now because of his illness. When she was old enough to walk, he took her everywhere he went—to the grocery story, the lumberyard, to the seed store, everywhere.

There are two visions of them together that I recall vividly. It is as if the scenes are framed and hanging in our hallway so that I see them whenever I walk past. One scene is of a time when Carol was about two, or maybe three years old. It had snowed, and all day she had begged me to take her out to play in it.

"Wait until daddy gets home from work," I told her, "maybe he will take you outside."

It was already dark when he got home, but she had not forgotten about playing in the snow. After dinner she asked him, "Daddy will you help me make a 'toe' man?"

So, bundled in her little brown snowsuit, she and daddy went outside where he not only helped her make a snowman (a very small one), but he allowed her to make an angel figure of herself by lying with her arms outstretched in the snow.

Job has always been a very spiritual person and would naturally want his children to be as well. The other scene that stands out in my memory of father and daughter together arises out of this concern. After the birth of the children I seemed to be perpetually tired, and often on Sundays I didn't go to church. He always did, with Carol accompanying him.

On the Sunday that I see so clearly, she was all dressed and sitting on my lap waiting for 'daddy' to come out of our bedroom. She saw him coming down the hallway and ran to meet him. She took hold of his hand and said, "Come on, dad, let's go."

By the time Amy was born Job's job required that he work the night shift. With time spent commuting by train from job to home, he didn't get home until 1:30 in the morning, which was just the time that Amy would awaken for her feeding. He must have been very tired, because his work in the data processing unit of a large bank was very demanding.

But, while I slept, he would heat the baby's formula, change her diaper (we didn't have throwaway ones back then), and hold her until she finished her bottle. Sometimes during the process I would awaken and hear Job cooing to her to drink every last drop of formula, and gently urging her to give up the required after feeding burp.

TWENTY-SEVEN

Take it for a better reason.
Take it because the years are long,
And full of sharp wearing days
that wear out what we are and what we have been
and change us into people we do not know,
living among strangers.
Lest you and I who love
Should wake some morning strangers and
Enemies in an alien world, far off.
—Author Unknown

July 1, 2001 (Sunday)

Last night Job's behavior was so erratic, so absolutely crazy, that in addition to hiding the door keys, I hid the sharp knives, skewers, letter opener, scissors, and anything else with a point on it. He was in a frenzy of frantically packing clothes in bundles that he secured with his belts. He either filed or cut the "Safe Return" bracelet (used by Alzheimer's sufferers prone to wander) from his wrist, and there was nothing I could do to stop him. It had arrived by mail only a few days earlier.

This morning I was afraid to get out of bed. He was asleep and I didn't want to awaken him. I knew that as soon as I got up he would get up as well, and I didn't know what awful things he would do. He did just what I expected and woke up when I left the bed, but there was no sign of the agitated behavior of last night.

He dressed casually. I guess he doesn't realize that it is Sunday. I reminded him of the time we should leave home in order to make the 9:30 service. He changed into different clothing, but they were less his usual style of dress than the ones he had on previously. When I made no comment about either set of clothing, he changed and dressed with his usual elegance.

The congregation was standing for the portion of liturgy that begins the worship service when Job suddenly sat down and slumped over. Oh, dear God, I thought, what is happening. Some of the men helped me get him into our car and we came home. Job went right to bed and slept for about an hour. He got up and I prepared his lunch, and he acted as if nothing had happened. What caused the reaction that he had? I don't know.

He is losing his mind. I know it. He decided to go for a walk. This time I knew that he was going but the neighbors did not know that I knew. It was very comforting to see many of them rushing to tell me that Job was walking alone. What am I to do? He is too sane to go to a nursing home, and too ill for me to care for him alone. I simply cannot go on like this. I need to cry. I need to get away, and I can't do either. I am afraid, but I do not want to burden the children with my tales of woe.

This afternoon a storm came up and broke the heat wave that has been with us for the past three to five days. It is comfortable tonight. No fans are whirring. The air conditioner is also silent.

July 2, 2001 (Monday)

What a perfectly delicious day it is, the result of rain yesterday that broke the heat spell. I weeded one flowerbed. In the vegetable garden I staked the tomato plants, which are heavy with green tomatoes. Both are jobs that Job used to do by himself. Today he did help some and seemed very pleased that he was making a contribution to worthwhile projects.

We went to the library. The librarian obviously did not know of Job's memory problem, so I had to tell her. Job had been on the Library Board that was responsible for getting the library built and opened in time for the bicentennial in 1976. He was a very effective Board member. I believe that during the years he served, (and they were many), he was elected to every office necessary for the Board's functioning.

And he volunteered so many hours to library work, I sometimes felt like a "Library Board Member widow!" I was very proud of him though, and of the service he gave to the community.

He signed out a book today, but he won't read it. Before we left, the librarian gave me a big hug because she knew how active and intelligent Job had been, and that now he is a person of diminished capacity, and we are both saddened by that awful truth.

At home Job slept for about twenty minutes then said, "I think I'll go for my walk now."

"No," I told him rather emphatically, "you've taken off your Safe Return bracelet. If you go for a walk I will have to go with you, and I am too tired for that."

He got angry and went a little crazy. Actually, he went a lot crazy and hurled his usual accusation of "you think I'm dumb and stupid" at me. He was still angry when we sat down to dinner and continued to act in a way that he knew annoyed me. He mashed, and mashed his baked potato as if he were trying to puree it. He cut his piece of sliced tomato into tiny, tiny pieces and put it on a piece of cold toast left over from breakfast. He went into his obnoxious mode of breathing loudly and heavily, a behavior that always makes me nervous.

It's too much to write about. He was positively crazy, crazy, crazy.

Today has been beautiful. Flowers are blooming, flowerbeds are clean, there is a shimmering blue sky, and it is quasi-cold.

July 3, 2001 (Tuesday)

Oh, oh, phlox have started to open. In our yard they are the last of the summer flowers to bloom, and I equate their opening with the end of summer. Oh, sad goodbye to summer.

Amy is home. She came up (from Maryland) for a dental appointment. Daddy went to Doylestown with her to keep the appointment. I went to K-Mart and bought him a new razor like the one he has used for years. He insists that the one he got as a Christmas gift, refused to use for over a year, but has used grudgingly since I had it checked out at the repair shop, doesn't work properly.

We are all at home now and Amy is at the piano accompanying him as he plays his clarinet. The music sounds good. He still remembers his notes and how to play his instrument. I am so glad that he hasn't lost that talent. I realize that it is the short-term memory that goes first, but there is evidence that some memories of the past are beginning to slip away as well.

July 4, 2001 (Independence Day)
   There are no holiday celebrations on this end of our street, Apple Drive. Across the street my neighbor is mowing his lawn. The children of the neighbors on both sides of us have visited and left the home of their parents. Amy left for home at 1:30 leaving Job and me alone with a big chunk of day to fill.
   We went for a long walk. With that over we drove to Zany Brainy. I bought two small wading pools because next week we are having guests with small children. The pools will give them something to do. Our Esther Williams above-ground pool has been gone since 1995, and the swing sets, popular when our children were little, disappeared well before that.
   At home I tried unsuccessfully to set the clock on the VCR. It has been blinking for days. That was a job that Job would have done with ease. We watched the Public Broadcasting station news. When it was over at 7:00, Job decided that he wanted to go for a walk!
   "Absolutely not," I said. "You really must give some consideration to my health."
   He seemed to understand but sulked all the same. We ate supper. He washed up the dishes. We often sit in our bedroom to relax, and watch TV programs that are reasonably free of graphic sex scenes and violence. While we were watching Job became restless and got up and started moving about the room.
   He went to the closet and began taking clothes and shoes out of it.
   "Why are you doing that?" I asked him.
   "I'm getting things ready to take out of the house," he said. "Don't we have to take everything home?" he said.
   "We are at home," I explained, but he continued with what he was doing.
   He is getting impossible for me to deal with. Am I going to have to "put him away?" There is a gentleman at the fitness center who volunteers information to me frequently about a man who finally had to "put his wife away" after she inflicted knife wounds on herself, then came after him (her husband) with the knife.

Job's behavior is vexing and frustrating to me, but it is not threatening. Still, the toll that it is taking on my nervous system demands a remedy, but what?

July 5, 2001 (Thursday)
This is the first Thursday that Job has spent at Elder Care. He has been going on Tuesdays. It was good to be at home alone, but I did miss him. This is what it will be like if I outlive him, or if we must be separated for any reason, I thought.

With him out of the house for a while, I didn't get much rest. I was too busy rushing around trying to catch up on things left undone when he is under foot. When I picked him up at 4:00 he was glad to see me. There was a twinkle in his eyes and a smile on his lips reminiscent of bygone days when our eyes would meet across a crowded room.

July 6, 2001 (Friday)
Together, we got the housework done. Job ran the vacuum and dusted living and dining room. I did the laundry and Job hung it on the line outside. In the late afternoon we went to Peddlar's Village and used the gift certificate that Amy had given us at Christmas to have lunch at restaurant there.

Job has been good all day.

July 7, 2001 (Saturday)
It was 7:00 when I awoke this morning. I was surprised to find Job's arm around me—like old times. It hardly happens anymore. All day he has been so rational it is frightening. It started last night. We played piano and clarinet duets together.

Today after fitness center we went to IHOP for breakfast. It was almost 11:00 when we got home. After a trip to inspect the garden, Job fell asleep and slept until I awoke him at 2:30. He is calm and in conversation responds pleasantly.

Thank you, God.

July 8, 2001 (Sunday)
I could have predicted that today would be a bad one. I had to help Job with a couple of decisions as he was getting dressed and he accused me of "picking on him." I reminded him that he

hadn't shaved. It is not something that I choose to do battle over. I simply knew that in the past he would have shaved. But that was then; this is now.

July 9, 2001 (Monday)
The weather is still agreeable. The sun is shining. There is no humidity. Mark (our son) has been dead for thirty-nine years today.

July 12, 2001 (Thursday)
Morning shadows are lengthening. It was 6:30 before I awoke. In the evenings the weather feels more like fall than early summer. Job stayed a few hours at Elder Care, so I was able to get a bit of work done but didn't get any rest.

Job seemed very happy to see me when I picked him up, but he didn't utter a single word during the fifteen or twenty minutes it takes for us to get home. The only time he tries to make conversation is if we are in a long line of traffic. Then, he will say, "Boy, I wonder where all that traffic came from."

He always goes right to the kitchen and starts looking into whatever pots or pans I have on the stove.

I know that I asked in a kindly voice if he had washed his hands after being in a public place. He said that he had, but I know that he hadn't. Just my asking made him angry, but I merely served up his plate and left him to eat alone while I went into our bedroom and sat down to relax.

July 14, 2001 (Saturday)
I didn't even ask Job to take off one of the two short-sleeved shirts he wore to the fitness center. Nor did I ask him to remove his tie. I did ask Michael, an attendant, if he would try to persuade him to remove the tie and one shirt. He took the tie off but kept the two shirts on all day. I 'm sure he expected me to comment but I didn't, thus avoiding a hassle.

Cicadas arrived today. After breakfast I sat on the patio for a long time listening to them sing. They sang only briefly. It is a beautiful day with temperate weather. The sky is very blue, with lots of clouds spread randomly over it. There is a large smoky gray one that occasionally obscures the sun for a long time. It feels chilly when this happens.

I am reading A Tree Grows in Brooklyn for the third time. I reread it every few years and always enjoy it.

July 16, 2001 (Monday)

I try to keep Job from wearing his good suits every day, but if they are left hanging in our closet he grabs one to put on no matter what work he engages in for the day. I store them in Amy's closet since she is no longer home to use it. He must have wandered into the room and saw them there. Last night, after cursing me out, he went into Amy's room to sleep. I don't know why he did that unless he saw his suits in the closet and figured that he was supposed to be there also. I don't remember what I did to provoke the vitriol, I just know that one of his "go-to-hells," "dammits," "I-don't-give-a-damns," came hurtling at me. Even though it is not the true personality of the Job that I married, it still hurts when he does this like salt in an open wound.

Where do these swear words come from? He never ever used such language before.

It might seem that I would have rested well with him not in bed with me, but I didn't. I hardly slept at all.

July 19, 2001 (Thursday)

Job had an appointment with the neurologist. The visits never last very long, just long enough for him to greet us and ask Job how he has been doing. Job always says he has been doing well, so I am the one who must give the doctor an accurate assessment of how I see the progression of Alzheimer's.

After the initial greeting the neurologist and Job go into another room where the doctor administers a test then makes his own determination of Job's condition. They come back to where I have been waiting and the doctor and I confer. I told him that I didn't believe the newest medicine we had tried was at all effective and that I preferred to go back to the Aricept he had prescribed originally.

July 21 through 23, 2001 (Saturday, Sunday, Monday)

On the spur of the moment I decided to drive to Maryland and visit Amy and James. The drive down was pleasant. We went to church with her on Sunday. We left to come home right after church, not even staying to have dinner with them. It is very warm today (Monday). I had to put the air conditioner on.

July 24, 2001 (Tuesday)

I had planned to leave Job at Elder Care for half a day, but when we came from the fitness center he said he didn't feel well. I encouraged him to lie down for a while and he did, but after lying down for less than an hour, he got up and got dressed. I am suspicious that the whole thing was a ruse to keep from going to Elder Care.

On this the hottest day of the year so far, in the very middle of the day he went outside to do weeding. He is jumpy and nervous. He is confused and uncooperative. It is maddening.

July 25, 2001 (Wednesday)

It is still hot but relief is forecast to come tonight. Job is restless. We went to the supermarket. I want to cry but tears won't come. Maybe they are hiding somewhere wondering why I need them. After all, I have not been injured. The children are well. No one close to me has died. Someone has died, but since the tears have not seen an inert body they do not know that a death has occurred.

July 26, 2001 (Thursday)

When I picked Job up from Elder Care he said he had had a bad day. He couldn't tell me what had made it bad. It has been cloudy all day. Days like this are hard on him. I've tried to keep him in a good mood but I can't.

July 27, 2001 (Friday)

It is almost 2:00. I am taking advantage of a beautiful day to sit on the patio and listen to cicadas sing. Job is inside in a dark, dark mood.

July 29, 2001 (Sunday)

Mom has been dead thirty-eight years today. I never told her that Carol was on the way. It was not the kind of thing that I felt comfortable talking to her about. I think she knew anyway.

July 31, 2001 (Tuesday)

Job and I played a piano/clarinet duet after dinner. I have tried to find someone who plays piano to come in and accompany him. I can do it but if someone else would it would give him an opportunity to socialize with a person other than me, and give me a break from caregiving.

Earlier in the day he had asked if we were going back down to Harry's. Harry was his brother. He died in 1993.

August 1, 2001 (Wednesday)

Crickets have not appeared yet, but cicadas still sing. We have had a lovely day of sunshine without oppressive heat. I've not done much today. After dinner Job and I went to Dairy Queen and had an ice cream sundae. It was a nice outing, although I would have preferred that he not have worn a long-sleeved, winter weight shirt.

After we were in bed, Job moved his head very close to mine. It was as if he could not get his head close enough to the space between my head and shoulders where it had rested contentedly so many times before. I caught a tiny glimpse of yesterday.

TWENTY-EIGHT

Job HAS THE KIND OF FLESH that seems to hold heat. That may be characteristic of other men. I am familiar only with Job's. Since body heat adjusts to weather temperatures, I did not notice this feature about him in the cold month of February when we were married.

When warmer months came I found that the place on his bosom where I always placed my head for sleeping was not comfortable to touch because it was so warm. Once when he was sleeping I went into the bathroom, wet a wash cloth with cold water, carried it into the bedroom and laid it on his chest.

"Ouch, What are you doing?" he exclaimed.

"Just cooling a place to lay my head," I calmly answered.

The prank gave a boost to his ego, I'm sure, and he accepted it with good humor, but I knew it was the kind of stunt that only a new bride could get away with without fear of recrimination.

August 2, 2001 (Thursday)

They told me at Elder Care that Job had done fine all day but at one point did ask if he could "call his wife." Good. That let's me know that he still knows that I am his wife.

August 8, 2001 (Wednesday)

After church Sunday we drove to the city to visit the house where Paul Robeson lived out his final days in the home of his sister, Marion Forsythe. Standing in the place where he had lived moved me almost to tears. I've always admired his genius. I seemed to feel his presence in the room.

On Monday we went to the Naval Air Station and filled out

papers to see if Job can get help with his prescription drugs through the Veterans Administration.

I must consider leaving him at Elder Care two full days instead of two half days. The half days give me time to do a few errands but no time to rest.

It is still very hot. Today's temperature reached one hundred degrees. We stayed inside all day after our trip to the supermarket. Glen and Patricia Nolan from church visited us. Job didn't contribute much to conversation, but he was really pleased about their visit.

August 9, 2001 (Thursday)

It's Betty's birthday. She's seventy-three. It always seemed strange that she is my niece, yet she is a month older than I am. In a month I will catch up with her. It has been hot and humid all day. The temperature went to one hundred degrees. It was almost unbearable. Some couldn't bear it and died, newscasters reported.

While Job was at Elder Care I had lunch with a friend that I hadn't seen since middle (Junior High) school days fifty-seven years ago. I couldn't have picked her out in a crowd and knew her only because I was expecting her. The drug store where we met was not crowded. She arrived at the time we had set. After we sat down to lunch she admitted that in a crowd she would not have recognized me either.

Her hair was a yellowish gray. It looked stiff and lacquered. She appeared well enough but said the doctor has told her that she has a dementia but it is not Alzheimer's.

It is not even 7:00 and Job is already in bed. I pleaded with him to get up, as he will only get up later and go wandering about. He wouldn't get up.

As I write, I am sitting at the little round picnic table that we've placed in the middle of the spot where the swimming pool stood. Once in a while a breeze wafts by gently. Cicadas are singing, and there is the eternal dull drone of airplanes revving up at the Air Station. The constant humming of traffic moving along County Line Road and that on Route 611 can be heard. Crickets have started to chirp now that it is getting darker.

It is coming up to 9:00. A light is on in the bathroom. I guess

Job is getting bathed so that he can get dressed and "go to work."

August 10, 2001 (Friday)
   It is still very hot. News broadcasters have warned elderly people, and young children to be careful because of it. Job put on a jacket, and luckily, a sun hat and announced that he was going for a walk. Without argument, I let him. By midday, clouds came, and still later, rain. It is somewhat cooler but humidity is still high, and I still need the air conditioner to be on.
   Job is packing things up again. I've asked him repeatedly not to. Finally I put everything away and told him very emphatically not to take them out again.

August 11, 2001 (Saturday)
   Ah, finally, relief from the oppressive six-day heat wave has come. Just when I thought the day would go right, it went all wrong. Job got out of bed ready to pack things. I wrote notes of what we would be doing during the day and posted them where it was impossible for him not to see, but he claimed he didn't see them. On our drive to the fitness center he said he had chest pains. He didn't exercise. I did.
   All day he insisted on packing things up. We argued. He complained that he was cold and kept closing windows as fast as I opened them. I brought him a blanket and a robe. He already had on a jacket. It was very stressful for me, but I held my ground. It has not been a pleasant day.

August 14, 2001 (Tuesday)
   While Job was at Elder Care, his sister Gwen called. She rarely does. We talked longer than we have since I've known her.
   After dinner, Job washed the dishes. He seemed tired, and was stumbling about. He was out of breath. I wonder what they do to him at Elder Care. He seems okay now and is reading the paper.

August 28, 2001 (Tuesday)
   Job didn't go with me to the fitness center. He said that he was tired. Several of the regulars asked me where he was. They always do now that they know of his illness. After breakfast we

went to Sesame Place. Julian had fun. Mostly, I was hot and tired. Crowds of people were there, wringing out the last bit of summer fun before school starts and vacations are over.

After his initial morning interlude of not feeling well, Job has been good. He has been more cheerful than usual. Maybe playing with Julian boosted his morale.

Crickets are keeping up a steady chorus outside. Otherwise, the night is still. Quiet. No cars pass. Only crickets are active, singing August away.

August 29, 2001 (Wednesday)

I should have enjoyed this day but I didn't. The weather is perfect. It is clear, with scattered clouds that look like boats sailing in the sky. I had typed Marty's Morning Friends' class list and lost it because the disc to my word processor didn't work. It is almost ten years old. Job bought it for me as a Christmas gift. I went to Marty's house and redid the list on Bob's laptop computer. Tomorrow I will go over and type the list for her afternoon class.

With Carol at home with us we sit up late watching TV shows from the seventies—Andy Griffith, and others. Carol takes daddy with her wherever she goes, so by nighttime he is tired and sleeps well. He even sleeps a wee bit longer than usual in the mornings.

August 30, 2001 (Thursday)

Where did August go? It seems to have gone before it arrived. There was no time to even reminisce about August revival meetings that were held in Black churches throughout our little town in South Carolina when I was growing up. Family members who had migrated to cities like Philadelphia, New York, Chicago, and Detroit, in search of jobs came home for revival meetings.

Most days, thoughts of Job crowded out all others. There were no spare moments for remembering other times. There was no time to think of anything except how tired I always am, and how sick Job is. Carol carried the children for a ride on the train. Julian loves to play with toy trains and to ride in real ones.

August 31, 2001 (Friday)

Job went with Carol and the children to New Jersey to visit

her cousin, his niece, Karen. I didn't prepare any dinner as I was sure she would see that daddy ate before coming home. None of them had eaten dinner. She brought home a pizza.

I enjoyed being home alone. I read parts of Kathryn Graham's book.

September 1, 2001 (Saturday)

Early in the morning we left for Bethany Beach, Delaware. We stayed in a wonderful beach house that overlooked a canal. A few boats were moored in the greenish colored water. It was great having the family together. Karen drove my car so that I wouldn't have to, Aaron came from Cincinnati, and on our way to the beach we picked him up at the airport and he rode down with us. Amy and James joined us on Monday.

On Sunday we drove down to Assateague Park, Maryland to see wild horses. There's a story about the horses but I need to look at my park circulars to know what it is, and I don't remember where I put the circulars. We only saw one or two horses from afar. Luckily, we had our car radios on and were informed that the park was closed.

All of us went to the beach every day. I thought it was ambitious of Carol to take little Alana, but both she and the baby handled it well. We saw dolphins playing in the water. Julian had fun playing in the sand and being carried into the water by his mom, dad, Cousin Karen, or Aunt Amy.

At night we played games. One that we enjoyed very much was called "Cranium." Aaron and Karen played partners and were the winners.

Saturday, the eighth, was our final day in the rented beach house. We all ate breakfast together in that lovely setting. I said the table Grace and added a prayer that we would all get home safely.

Aaron and Carol called from the hotel where they stopped before continuing on to Cincinnati. She called again when they arrived at home on Sunday.

On Sunday I started to feel sad again. Job is as he was before. He started in again right away to being cantankerous.

September 10, 2001 (Monday)

We spent the day doing a few errands. At night Job went to

bed at 8:00. Later at night, of course, he attempted several times to get up and "go to work." His attitude toward me is very bad. I am making a desperate, desperate effort to stay calm and let him know that I care about him. I try to make conversation. His responses are usually caustic, and rarely follow up on the topic I introduced. He doesn't act the same when other people are around as he does when just he and I are together.

September 11, 2001 (Tuesday)

Oh, fateful, fateful day. The television is always on at the fitness center. That's where we were when the terrorists attacked the Twin Towers in New York. The Center was filled with men and women working out on various pieces of equipment. Everyone was of the opinion when the first building was hit that it was a terrible, terrible accident. When the second building was hit, without consulting with one another, all of us recognized the deed for what it was.

I don't remember when I heard of the car bomb going off at the State Department. When we got home, news of the attack on the Pentagon was being broadcast, as well of the plane that was downed in Western Pennsylvania.

Each time it was mentioned on the many news broadcasts over the several days that it was the main news story, I would explain to Job what it was all about. But no matter how many times I repeated it, he wouldn't remember, and the rest of us will never forget.

September 12, 2001 (Wednesday)

The news all day has been about the tragedy that happened in downtown Manhattan New York, Washington, D.C., and Western Pennsylvania yesterday. The thing that stays constantly on my mind is that I will never, never feel safe in this country again.

Leaves are slowly starting to fall from their spring and summer home. Mornings are chilly but hot weather comes later in the day. When I picked Job up from Elder Care he was interacting with a group of other senior clients. He was talking, and smiling, and didn't come to where I was waiting for him even though he knew that I was there.

September 15, 2001 (Saturday)

Talk of the terrorist attack is slowly waning, and no longer dominates news reporting.

At the fitness center, Job worked out on all of his prescribed pieces of equipment. At home during the day he worked fever-ishly raking up crabapples from the driveway and front lawn. When night came I thought he would surely be tired enough to sleep through the night. He was in bed by 8:30, but by 9:30 was up again.

He took a shower and dressed himself for going to church even though I told him that it was Saturday night. He continued his preparations for going out. When I knew that he was not going to change his mind, I decided to ignore him, thinking that he would go to the door, see that it was dark, and come back inside. He didn't. He went out into the night. I called and called to him to come inside, and when he didn't, I went out and some-how, I don't know how, convinced him to come back inside.

September 16, 2001 (Sunday)

It is starting again, that urge, but inability to weep. I felt it when we came from our trip to Bethany Beach, but strangely, not after the disaster of this past Tuesday. It is starting to hit me now. I look out over our freshly mowed lawn, and up at the sun shin-ing from a cloudless blue sky, and I think, five thousand lives, ten thousand pairs of eyes, through no fault of their own, will never again see such a day as this.

Amy works in Washington. She is so afraid. We all are afraid.

September 20, 2001 (Thursday)

I am actually sitting down doing absolutely nothing. On Monday Carol chided me for never taking time to relax. Job is at Elder Care. I no longer feel guilty about leaving him there for two full days, even though it takes a larger bite out of our savings than I would like.

It wasn't a day that he was to go to Elder Care, so yesterday he worked all day raking crabapples from the front lawn and from the driveway. After dinner he went out and continued working. I went downstairs to watch the news and forgot to check on his whereabouts. I grew concerned when full daylight turned to dusk and he hadn't come inside.

I called and called to him but he didn't answer. I knocked on the door of my neighbor with whom he occasionally visits. He was not there. I got in the car and drove around the neighborhood and didn't see him. I was on the phone with 911 giving a description of him when the daughter of our other next door neighbor knocked on our door.

"Mrs. Winters," she said, "Mr. Winters is in our house drinking a glass of ginger ale. He said you didn't know where he was."

"Thank you, Brenda," I said, and went to their door and asked him if he would please come home now.

It wasn't that I minded that he visited, but I felt that he should have let me know that he was going. Along with the relief of discovering that he had not wandered into the next little town contiguous to ours was a desire to inflict some mild bodily harm that would let him know how distressed I was when I couldn't find him.

September 24, 2001 (Monday)

Job started the day off in a crying mood. I wanted to make apple jelly and got up at 7:00 to get started with that endeavor. I encouraged Job to stay in bed a while longer, but he got up, got dressed, and came into the kitchen and ate a bowl of cereal.

It is still quite warm, and our windows and doors are left open during the day. When he discovered that the house was open, he feigned sickness, put his pajamas back on, and went back to bed. He stayed there for about half an hour, then got up again in a more cheerful mood. He has worked in the yard quite a bit today. It is encouraging to see him take the initiative to do something!

September 25, 2001 (Tuesday)

Dear Julian, my precious little grandson. You gave me this journal for Christmas, 2000. Aunt Amy had given me one the year before, so I used hers first. Maybe some day you will read what I am writing and know that you had a grandmother who loved you very much.

This past summer I had a chance to spend a week with you, your mom and dad, and your little sister, "Wanna." We had a wonderful time. It was fun watching you play in the water and in the sand. Uncle James helped you make sandcastles.

Americans are still sad about the tragedy of September Eleventh, and because of a possible impending war.

September 27, 2001 (Thursday)

The magic day has arrived, my seventy-third birthday. I'm okay with it. I received beautiful cards from Carol, Julian, and Alana. I didn't get one from Job but he has given me so many beautiful ones in the past, I don't hold this year's lack against him. On Saturday we are going to visit Amy and James. I'm sure there will be a card from her waiting for me when I arrive.

September 29, 2001 (Sunday)

In addition to the card, James had bought a birthday cake for me. After dinner they sang Happy Birthday to me, and we ate ice cream and cake. Amy had taken Job to a store and he bought me a beautiful, beautiful card. I know he made the selection himself. No matter which of us a card is for, he always insists on making his own selection.

October 13, 2001 (Saturday)

I hate to see all of the apples from our three producing trees go to waste. I've canned some, made jelly and applesauce, and given away some to whoever would take them. This afternoon my niece, Gwendolyn, came to pick some.

Things between Job and me have been bad all day. There are some things I simply refuse to let him get away with and blame on Alzheimer's. By nightfall his behavior was such that I had to call Carol and have her talk to him. She was able to calm him down. I was too tired to lie awake worrying about it, so I slept soundly throughout the night.

October 14, 2001 (Sunday)

Things were much better today. We went to church. Lately Job has found reasons to weep silently during some part of the service. Today, I felt he was being repentant for his perfectly awful behavior yesterday.

October 22, 2001 (Monday)

Job's days continue to alternate between good and bad. Mostly they are bad, in that he gives me lots of grief. Getting him to bathe and change underwear are the usual bones of contention. Getting him to remove his dirty (sometimes two days worth of dirty) clothes are times when he is likely to tell me to "go to hell, he's not a child for me to tell him what to do."

He is doing an excellent job of raking leaves, but there is still a generous amount to be raked up.

I've spent a great deal of time today trying to find places for books that I will not use again but hate to throw away. I still feel lonely, and am still searching for some meaning to my life.

In the back, our neighbor's dog is barking a deep, hoarse bark. There are no other sounds in the development.

October 23, 2001 (Wednesday)

Some days I do not record anything in my journal because I am too tired. Tonight I have time and am not overly tired, but what is there to write about except the weather? It felt like summer all day. The temperature climbed to ninety-three degrees, setting a one hundred-year record for this date.

I was up before Job. I like that, as I can enjoy a quiet cup of coffee and scan the newspaper before beginning the day's activities. Sometimes I must wait until after he goes to sleep at night before tackling the "jumble" and "cryptogram."

He had an appointment with the ophthalmologist. In the office he had a small, or rather, a fairly large fit. It started with his characteristic trembling, a behavior that I have learned to ignore. He does it when we are riding in the car. First, he looks to see where the heat gauge is set. If he thinks that it is on a setting that doesn't produce heat, he begins to tremble. I have put a blanket in the car and when he complains I tell him to cover himself with it. Often he does, wrapping himself from his neck down to his feet. When he gets too warm, he starts to gasp for breath.

When I ignored the trembling in the ophthalmologist's office, he doubled up with trembling, and finally toppled onto the floor.

"Get up, Job," I encouraged, I'm afraid, using a less than a pleasant tone. He raised his voice in anger.

"Don't you think I'm trying to get up? I'm cold, cold, cold, dammit, and nobody cares."

Seeing him rolling around on the floor, a nurse came and spoke very compassionately to him.

"Mr. Winters would you like to move to another office where it is not so cold?" she asked.

She did take us to a different spot. I couldn't see that the temperature was more comfortable than where we had been, but her psychology worked. Job had gotten the attention he wanted, and he settled down to wait his turn to be examined.

All day, he has done little things to try to provoke me to an argument. I have quietly ignored him and have offered no resistance to anything he has done, no matter how eccentric it was. About an hour ago he started rushing around frantically, looking for—what? I never know. He has dressed himself in two shirts to go out. He had on a jacket and cap for going outside. He has taken them off and is sitting in his recliner holding a bed pillow.

Days, he gives me grief. Nights, he gives me grief. I fear I will have a stroke, so that even if I outlive him, I will know no further peace or moments of happiness in this life.

October 28, 2001 (Sunday)

Clocks were reset last night, reflecting the end of daylight saving time. Job has acted quasi-sensibly all day. I have refused to allow his contrary behavior to get me bogged down in conflict. Right now he is getting dressed for going to bed. He has put on one of his daytime shirts to sleep in although there is a clean pair of pajamas hanging in the closet where he can see them.

When he first started to do that I tried to reason with him that it made extra work for me, as I try to keep his clothes clean. Now, I don't say anything when he does it. Oops, seeing that I am not going to challenge him, he has taken off the shirt. I'll see if he puts his underwear back on or decides on the pajamas.

October 31, 2001 (Wednesday)

Job has been good all day. We cleaned the front and back gutters of leaves that had collected in them. We drove down to the Mall. After dinner we watched "Dial M for Murder" for the zillionth time.

On days like this, when he is agreeable, it makes me sad to contemplate that some day we may be separated because of his illness. I would miss him more than I care to think about.

November 7, 2001 (Saturday)

We spent the weekend with Amy and James. Carol, Aaron, and the children came from Ohio, and we were all together as a family again. That always makes me happy.

We had an enjoyable day together. I don't know what triggered it, but while he was in the bathroom getting ready for bed, Job began crying and talking to himself, asking God to "Please take him Home." I was already in bed and didn't get up to investigate the behavior, as I have become acquainted with it.

Amy knocked on the bathroom door and asked if he was all right. He told her that he was. Eventually he came to bed.

AMY IS THE DAUGHTER THAT HAS SHOWN QUIET CONCERN for 'daddy'. The cards she chooses for her father's birthday and Fathers' Day always express a sentiment of appreciation for his guidance, understanding, and love. Carol, on the other hand, usually chooses one that is at least semi-humorous.

During the time of his volunteer work with the library, he was often called to investigate when the alarm in the building sounded. The calls came at night after the library had closed. The policy was that before answering the call, Job was to call the Township police and ask them to meet him there. One night the alarm sounded twice. The first time, Job called the police to meet him. When the alarm went off the second time shortly after he had returned from the first sounding, he did not call the police.

I begged him to call and became angry when he didn't.

"OK," I said. "If you don't call the police I am not going to either."

But my declared unconcern did not lessen the anxiety I felt about his going into an unknown situation. Amy was downstairs watching television. I ran down to tell her about her father. Without comment, and without hesitation, she came upstairs and went to the telephone.

"Hello," I heard her say, "This is Amy Winters. My father has just left home to investigate why the alarm went off at the library.

Will you please meet him there?"

November 24, 2001 (Saturday)
I continue to leave Job at Elder Care for five hours two days a week. Some days I think I'll leave him for only four hours to keep from having to pay for a full day. But I've come to realize that I really need the few hours of freedom that leaving him at Elder Care allows me.

The children are still visiting for the Thanksgiving holiday. Julian and his uncle James are sitting at the kitchen table having fun with play dough. Job is sitting there also, but although Julian begs him to, he doesn't join in playing with him.

Job and Amy did play piano/clarinet duets earlier. It is heart-warming that he still does extremely well with his music.

The children are leaving for home later tonight. It seems a long time since just Job and I were at home together alone. This morning he was very difficult, refusing to dress properly. I was glad that Carol was here to observe his behavior that I try to tell her about by telephone.

November 29, 2001 (Thursday)
The month has only one day left to spend. Then, it will have used up its allotment for the year. Days and weeks have wings, which they use very efficiently to whisk them away to eternity.

November days are often gray and dreary. Today, with drizzling rain, is such a day. I left Job at Elder Care while I did a few errands. Since I finished them early, I decided to pick him up before the full complement of hours were used up. I thought he would express gratitude that he was in his own home earlier than he had expected to be. He didn't.

He went straight away to the kitchen and tried to prepare dinner. An hour passed before he realized that he wouldn't be able to. He came into the bedroom and asked if I would come and help him. Does it seem cruel that I said no? Walking in my shoes one would understand my refusal. I said further that I would not enter the kitchen at all until he came out with the intention of staying out until I called him in to dinner.

He has given me a hard time all day. Nothing big. Little things, like slowing around unnecessarily when accomplishing simple tasks. I am angry, my stomach is in knots.

I am in bed and hope that reading, along with eating one of the "wollypops" that I bought for Julian, will help me to relax.

December 5 through 24, 2001

It is warm enough that I felt comfortable sitting outside to eat lunch. Lawn chairs have been put away for the winter. I carried a kitchen chair outside and sat at a table that is left there covered. Job elected not to join me, but ate sitting at the kitchen table. This is the perfect weather for enjoying eating out of doors. In late spring it is often too chilly, and in the summertime, dodging intrusive yellow jackets presents a daunting challenge.

Carol has called and given me some good news. Aaron has found a job in Virginia and they will be relocating there. While they were visiting Amy and James he felt nostalgic for his native Maryland. That works out well for Carol who has wanted to move closer to us so that she can visit more often and lend a helping hand with daddy. Amy has been good about coming up to help as often as she can.

I feel a little happy and a little sad about the move. I had gotten used to flying out to visit them. Of course, since September eleventh, I would not have flown again. I hope things work out for them in their new location.

We went by train to visit them a week before Christmas, then went from there to spend the holiday with Amy and James. Traveling with Job is so difficult I don't think I will attempt any more trips to anywhere. I carry as little luggage as possible, but the few things that must be hand carried still seem cumbersome.

Knowing of Job's frequent need to use toilet facilities, whenever we pass restrooms I always encourage him to go. He refuses, saying that he doesn't feel the need to do so. However, as soon as we are well beyond the facility, he needs to go. Since I must accompany him or he would get lost, it means taking the luggage back to what usually ends up being some distance away.

It is Christmas Eve. Amy and James met us at Washington's Union station. We are in their home now. I did very little Christmas shopping, choosing rather to give the children a sum of money to spend as they wish. I hope Amy will use hers to purchase a lawn mowing service for the summer, and that Carol will buy a freezer with hers.

December 25, 2001 (Tuesday–Christmas Day)

In one hour and fifty minutes from now Christmas Two Thousand and One, still not seeming like Christmas, will be history. None of us went outside all day. Lawns between houses in this upper middle class development are spacious, so we heard no movement, not even cars passing, throughout the day.

Amy's in-laws arrived at four, the time she had scheduled dinner. She had prepared a delicious dinner of roast beef, grilled salmon, broccoli, mashed white potatoes, a green salad, and freshly baked rolls. Sandy, her mother-in-law, always brings a fruit salad.

We had a choice of desserts: pecan, sweet potato, or mince meat pie, ice cream, or any combination of choices, all served with coffee or tea.

Carol called, wished us all a Merry Christmas, and said they liked the gifts they received from us. We opened gifts. Everyone liked the presents they were given. I was amazed at what thoughtful and practical gifts the children chose for us without spending a lot of money on items we would have little use for.

We have been away from home for a long time, almost two weeks, and I will be glad to get home even though I must resume the lonely and exacting job of caring for Job.

December 28, 2001 (Friday)

Amy and James had spent a few days with us. They left about an hour and a half ago. I was both glad and sorry that Amy got a chance to see her father in a light that I have come to see him often, yelling and cursing. I don't remember what precipitated the scene.

I was afraid that I would not be able to say goodbye without a flow of tears, but I did. They waited until later to come.

December 30, 2001 (Sunday)

The sun is shining, but it is cold. The wind blows slightly. We got up early, and both of us were dressed for going to church. Job began to act strangely. He sat in his recliner with his head bowed, not speaking. When I asked if he felt up to going to church, he said he didn't know what he wanted to do.

I didn't question him further, but later I mentioned that we might go to another church where the service started later than at ours. We still had time to make it if he wanted to go. He didn't respond at all, just sat.

After a while, he said he was going for a walk. I offered no objection to that, but as I've come to do of late when I am too tired to walk with him, I followed at a distance in the car. Still later, he walked for a long time in our back yard, picking up the many twigs that have fallen since winter began.

Once inside, he sat on the end of the sofa with his head down and his eyes closed. He appeared to be asleep, but not in a deep sleep. Occasionally he twitched as if he were having a seizure. He often does this, but when I ask him why, he says he doesn't know why.

Today, I think I have a full understanding of what it must be like to be a widow, living all alone.

December 31, 2001 (Monday)

When I awoke this morning Job had an arm around me. Perhaps he had a clear moment of remembering something of past years. As I lay with my back in the contour of his body, he began whispering words of endearment, and although I did not become emotionally involved, he somehow found that release of tension that men seek. Then, he slept. I hoped that the experience signaled some stabilizing quality of his mental decline.

Did he sense that today is the very last one of the year, and thus an appropriate one in which to try to get across a message to me that he still cared? As the day progressed, I came to realize that my "hope" was merely a futile mental exercise. Nothing of his disposition that has been caused by Alzheimer's dementia will ever revert to being normal.

TWENTY-NINE

BEFORE THE DEMENTIA JOB'S DISPOSITION was such that everyone who knew him either socially or at his place of employment, loved, or at least liked him. It always brought a smile to his face whenever I would say that to him.

"Why is it," I would ask, "that everybody loves you and nobody even likes me?"

"I guess it's because I'm such a lovable person," he would reply, adding, "besides, who said nobody likes you? I know plenty of people who like you."

He would continue, saying, "And even if nobody else likes you, I love you and that's all that really matters." It is a dialog that we've had many times during our years of marriage.

During the past two decades he has made many more visits to our family doctor's office than I have, as I have usually only gone into the office twice a year for regular checkups. Whenever I go, Dr. Miles never fails to ask, "How's Job?" So, when Job comes home from an office visit, I ask, "Did the doctor ask you about me?" He finds that amusing and replies while slightly blushing, and with what I've found to be a winning smile, "No, I'm afraid not."

There is another running question that over the years I have often put to Job.

"Job," I must have asked at least five times during each of the four decades since our wedding, "why did you choose to marry me? I know there were other girls who would have loved to have had you for their husband."

His answer after each query has been consistent. "I married you because I loved you. I still do."

"Why?" has been my next question.

"Because I saw in you all the qualities I wanted in a wife," has been his answer.

I accept his statements as truth, knowing that I can return the compliment to him. I like that he was (and is) clean-cut, highly intelligent, gentle yet manly. I like that he speaks well, that he has and has demonstrated great leadership skills. I like that during these forty-five years of marriage he has kept his promise to me to give me "all of the things I needed, and some of the things I wanted."

In order to keep his promise to provide me with the material things I needed, he worked very hard. At the time of our marriage he was a presser of clothes for rich families who lived on the Main Line. He was not unhappy with this menial job. He took great pride in doing his job well. I was not ashamed of his work, but I agreed with the slogan of the United Negro College Fund that "A mind is a terrible thing to waste." I worked for the federal government and encouraged him to at least take the Civil Service test for that work.

Admittedly, working as a clerk for the government would not elevate him to a higher level of prestige, but I felt that it could be a stepping stone to something better. And indeed it was. He now had time to pursue studies in other fields, and luckily he chose data processing. It was not then the big industry that it became later.

Civil Service did not extend the time of the temporary position he was hired to fill, and certainly, up to that time of his life, that was probably the greatest good fortune that could have befallen him. He didn't really have the temperament to be a government worker.

At the time that his Civil Service job ended I had just given birth to our first child. We also had only recently moved from our row house duplex in the city to our ranch home in the suburbs. After a short time of job-hunting, Job was hired to work in the Data Processing department of a large bank. On merit alone, he advanced to a level where he held a very responsible position.

Job loved his family so much. Every year he saw to it that we went on a vacation, even if only for a few days. And the vacation had to be far away enough that it meant staying overnight in a motel, because that is what the children enjoyed most. From the lower grades through high school, he attended every program that each child was part of.

And the years kept flying by without strife as our little family lived happily together.

In the early nineteen eighties Job suffered a heart attack which led to his undergoing by-pass surgery on a single artery. After a reasonable period of recuperation he was back at work, and I stood guard over him night and day looking for any signs of unfavorable consequences resulting from the heart attack.

At night, if he breathed so softly that I couldn't hear him I would call quietly to him.

"Job, are you asleep?"

"Um huh," he would answer. His reassurance didn't prevent my repeating the query again. Once when I asked him if he was sleeping he answered sleepily, "No, but I would be if you would stop waking me up."

I was desperately concerned about his health after the heart attack. A few years afterwards his job offered retirement packages to employees based on a formula of chronological age and number of service years with the organization. Job met the eligibility requirements, and I urged him to take advantage of it.

"Why don't you take advantage of the opportunity to quit," I asked him.

"I can't," he replied quite calmly, "I've got to put my children through school."

"Through school" meant helping them pay for their college education. He and I worked together in order to do that, but I was so proud of him for feeling that the responsibility was his alone. He always gave our girls the understanding that he would pay for their undergraduate degrees; for degrees above that, they were on their own.

Now, YOU HAVE MET BOTH the Dr. Jekyll and Mister Hyde personalities of Job. Have I, in good journalistic style, shown both personalities clearly? There are a few more details that sharpen his physical appearance but nothing else that I can share about the inner person that made him so dear to me and to our children. His face, unlike mine, which is oval-shaped, is angular. He has long arms. In a shirt, he buys a fourteen and a half neck size. In long sleeved shirts, his arms would need two inches more than the standard thirty-two-inch length usually used by manufacturers to accommodate that neck size.

I feel the need to escape from behind the personal pronoun "I" that I've used when referring to myself. Beginning here, I become Myrna. It is not the name given to me by my mother. When I was a little girl she told me that the name she had chosen for me came from a story that she had read where the girl (or young lady) was a "good girl," and she hoped that I would be like that girl.

Not until this very writing did I consider that maybe it was meant to be a subliminal message to me. Perhaps she had in mind "good girl" as it is used in modern society to describe a female who preserves her virginal state until after marriage. My mother was forty-four years old when I was born, and I am sure would have been uncomfortable discussing sexual matters with me. She has been dead for more than thirty years now. Whatever she meant, I have always thought of her "hopes" as being "good" in every respect.

Myrna. The name means "Soft or Gentle," or "Beloved." It is an apt pseudonym, partly. I lay no claim to possessing the first attribute, since it would be immodest to both bestow upon myself and authenticate the attribution. I do not hesitate to affirm that from the day we exchanged wedding vows to the present, Job has loved me dearly.

THIRTY

❦

OW GRIEVOUS IT IS FOR ME to record the journal entries for this New Year, and it is in this year that my narrative will end. I will not record the entries of each day, only those showing how the beast is winning the battle over reason and sanity in Job's life. There may be brief mention of the joys I experience when time is spent with our children and grandchildren, but only if they are connected to something relating to Job's cognitive decline.

My whole being, from the end of last year to the beginning of this one, has been caught up in the frustration of dealing with Job. I've used the term "caught up in" rather than "devoted to" because that is the best term for describing the situation accurately.

I have expended every human condition, psychological, physical, mental, emotional, and, yes, even spiritual, trying as compassionately as I can to help him stay in a loving, family setting rather than move into a "facility." I have remained to him a devoted wife. Had I not felt a genuine sense of devotion, I would not have felt "caught up" in caring for him.

Does it seem that I have complained about insignificant things, like his not wanting to change dirty underclothes for clean ones? Probably it does.

Since March, I have participated in a telephone support group that includes three other women. All of us have agreed to be part of a study that is being done by a hospital in the region. We do not know each other except by telephone voice. The common thread between us is that our spouses have Alzheimer's disease. One woman's husband does not have Alzheimer's, but has had a series of mini-strokes, and the resulting dementia mimics that caused by Alzheimer's.

During one telephone meeting the question was asked, "what is the behavior that your husband does that causes you the most frustration?"

"Oh, God," the woman whose husband's dementia resulted from mini-strokes answered, "there is no one thing. It's a series of little things that build up, and build up, until you are ready to go crazy."

I say, "amen" to that. Also, the series of little things need not occur in the same day. With me, one day it might be the constant pacing. Another day it might be because I must spend time looking for something that he has misplaced, like the checkbook, which I now hide. There are no street corner mailboxes in our development. We are allowed to put outgoing letters in our mailboxes for the postman to pick up when he delivers mail to our house. Seeing outgoing mail in the box, Job will remove it from the box, open it, and lay it down almost anywhere. He once opened the envelope containing the check for his health insurance payment. Quite by accident I discovered what had happened just in time to mail it so that it would reach its destination on time.

Adding to the frustration of looking for things that he has misplaced, I now am exasperated when I have hidden items (like keys or knives) from him and forget where I have put them, and when I need to use them, the process of looking begins all over again.

I know that Job appreciates that I try to take care of him. He infrequently says so, even now, when cognitive ability is slipping rapidly away from him. He says that he doesn't know what he would do without me, and that he appreciates all the things I do for him. And he apologizes for being difficult at times. When he was first diagnosed with the disease, he understood that he had Alzheimer's and that it affected his memory. Now, he no longer recognizes that he has dementia that causes him to do things that he would not ordinarily do.

January 1, 2002 (Tuesday)

We were still up when the New Year came in. I am glad that unlike last New Year's Eve, Job stayed up with me to await the arrival of the New Year. This morning we slept a little later than we usually do. I was up before Job and sat alone to drink the one cup of coffee a day that I allow myself to have. With it, I ate toast with some of my homemade apple jelly. It is selfish, I guess, but I do enjoy having this little ceremony alone in the quiet of morning.

When Job got up I prepared his breakfast and got busy with the chores that I will do today. The day has begun bright and clear. Each New Year's Day when the day is such as this one is I always think of the hymn, "Hail to the Brightness of Zion's Glad Morning." It's one of those old-fashioned hymns that nobody sings anymore. I don't know what it means, but I can hear its melody on days like this.

Angie (my brother) called to wish me a Happy New Year.

"Thanks," I said, "but I don't see that in the picture."

I wasn't sure if he knew of Job's Alzheimer's and would not have mentioned it, but he told me that his sister-in-law has the disease. I wonder who told him about Job?

Job and I went for a drive and stopped in a furniture store to look at a kitchen set. Along the drive I tried to draw him into conversation, but he wouldn't contribute a single word.

We were almost home when he adjusted the setting of the car heater. It was set for "hot." I thought he was too warm, because he turned the switch to "cold."

"Are you too warm?" I asked.

"No, I'm cold," he said, "my stomach is cold. My whole body is cold."

"But you turned the heat off," I said.

That set him into his angry "I never do anything right" mode. The rest of my day was ruined. My stomach knotted up, and my throat constricted. So much for the beginning of a Happy New Year, I thought. It is night. Dinner and the News Hour are over. We are in bed.

January 2, 2002 (Wednesday)

Oh, drat, I've missed getting my linen calendar for the New Year. I've gone to several stores looking for one without success.

We food shopped, and when we got home. I prepared lunch. It was a good lunch: a tuna sandwich, a chocolate cupcake, a few chips, and a tangerine.

Job washed up the dishes used in preparing lunch. I went into our bedroom to sit and relax for a few moments.

Presently, I heard a great noise coming from the living room. It was Job, shouting at full lung capacity, "Hallelujah! Praise God." He talked of God's goodness to him and entreated His mercy. Over, and over, it went. I didn't go out to him. I didn't say anything. I stayed in our bedroom. There was an interval of five or ten minutes of quiet, then the performance was repeated. I thought he had succumbed to madness and would never again be the Job I knew and loved.

After a while, he came into the bedroom. Neither of us mentioned what had transpired forty-five minutes earlier. He seemed to be just fine, and we went to a furniture store and bought a table and chairs for the kitchen. The old set was worn and outdated generally.

It is only 9:30. Job is not asleep but he has started to silently mumble words too softly for me to comprehend.

January 5, 2002 (Saturday)

Our new kitchen table was delivered today. It is very nice but is less compact than I wanted it to be. The top sets on a pedestal that doesn't allow the four chairs to fit against it when the drop leaves are down.

We went to the fitness center. Job only finished exercising on one piece of equipment. He became so confused the technician let him sit and read a magazine. I no longer try to help him because he doesn't listen to me. He usually responds well to the attendants.

Christmas lights are still on in some houses. Why don't they face up to it? Christmas is over. When I took a walk outside in this forty-degree temperature weather, I noticed that daffodils are already peeking through the ground.

January 6, 2002 (Sunday)

We went to church but left just after the sermon was over. All through the service Job had sat with his head down and his eyes closed. His arm began to shake in a kind of tremor. It does that when he gets agitated. I whispered and asked him if he wanted to go home. He said that he did.

He was miserable to live with for the rest of the day and into the night. At 6:30, he went to bed. He got up to get dressed twice before 9:00. Each time, I coaxed him back to bed. When he got up a third time, I didn't plead with him not to get dressed. The doors were locked and he didn't have a key to get out. At 10:00 I went to bed. Needless to say, I couldn't sleep. He didn't come to bed until 2:00 in the morning.

The first snowfall of winter, a light one, came early in the evening.

January 9, 2002 (Wednesday)

Tomorrow is trash collection day. Bulk items can be placed to curbside, so I asked Job to help me carry our old table and chairs out to be hauled away. He helped willingly. We talked about how much we were enjoying our new set.

I was surprised when later I found him sitting in the living room looking very sad and dejected.

"Job," I asked, "what's the matter? Why are you suddenly looking so down?"

"Why are you giving away all of our furniture?" he wanted to know.

"What do you mean, 'all of our furniture?' I threw out the old kitchen set. We bought a new one, remember?" I answered.

"Well, did you ask anyone about it? Did you ask James and Harry?" He asked

"Job, please," I answered, "I saw no reason to ask your dead brothers if I could throw away junk that we have no further use for."

It didn't occur to me that he was serious, so I told him that if he wanted to keep the set he could drag it back from the curb and store it in the basement, but I wouldn't help him.

THE DISCARDED JUNK FURNITURE incident must have been the factor that triggered the behavior that is recorded in my next journal entry. I've used the word "triggered" because information circulated by the Alzheimer's Association suggests that when a Catastrophic Reaction occurs, try to determine what might have "triggered" it.

In 1991 when Job began taking the medicine that both the neurologist and I agreed was affecting him adversely, I called the manufacturer of the medicine. I still do not understand how, but somehow they are associated with the Alzheimer's Association National Office.

From that call I began to receive on a regular basis information from them and from the local chapter to which they ultimately referred me. The information covers many of the situations that an Alzheimer's caregiver is likely to experience. I would learn later, that like myself, many caregivers simply did not have the time to keep up with reading the information received from the Association, along with a myriad other papers that he or she is now forced to read and try to comprehend.

The operators at the Alzheimer's Association were courteous if not always helpful and invited me to call as often as I felt the need to do so. I did call from time to time. I especially wanted them to know how the medicine they manufactured affected my husband's sexual behavior. And at least once I called to ask what I should do if at 2:00 or 3:00 in the morning my husband became so unruly that I couldn't handle him. I have no relatives or close friends nearby, and no neighbor that I would want to bother at such an hour.

Their advice on that was that I should call the police. "They won't arrest him," I was told, they would help me get him calmed down, and make suggestions as to whether he should get further attention.

The Alzheimer's Association's slogan is, "Someone to Stand by You." I believe that is true, but there are times when one feels that they are not standing near enough to help in those very dark, dark moments when you need someone standing right beside you.

January 10, 2002 (Thursday)

I awoke around 2:30 in the morning and discovered that Job was not in bed. That was not unusual. He would often get up and go to the bathroom, but when he came back into the bedroom he had no clothes on. I knew then that he had bathed and would dress for the day.

The doors were locked. He couldn't get out of the house, so I lay very still, not allowing him to know that I was awake. My hope was that he would realize that it was still night and come back to bed. He didn't.

When I was sure that he was not looking in the direction of

the bed, I chanced a look at the clock radio on his nightstand. The time was 3:25. He was fully dressed and kept pacing back and forth from the bedroom to the kitchen. In the bedroom he opened and closed the drawers of his dresser for what seemed like an interminable number of times.

Once he came into the bedroom, walked over to my dresser, and stood looking into the mirror. I saw his reflection. He looked so drawn, so haggard, so about ready to fall down, I felt I had to speak to him. His shoulders drooped. His eyes looked glassy and sinister.

"Are you looking for your glasses?" I raised up and asked.

"I don't know what I want," he said and left the room.

I followed, carrying his eyeglasses. Except for the kitchen, no lights were on in the front part of the house, so I could not see him.

"Where are you, Job?" I called to him but he didn't answer.

I put the light on and found him sitting at the table in the dining room at the place where he would normally sit for dinner. As soon as the light was on he began to shout out to the limit of his vocal capacity.

"Get out! Get out of my house NOW," he yelled.

He screamed other unkind things about me, but they were not spoken so dramatically, so I cannot remember what they were. I remember, however, that (how could I ever forget!) the vitriol continued.

Twice he screamed, "If I had a gun I would SHOOOT you."

Oddly, I didn't feel afraid. Yet, maybe I was afraid, but was too afraid to realize that I was.

I remember the calm with which I asked, "Do you want me to leave now Job, In the middle of the night?"

"YEEES, dammit. I want to be FREEEE! I. Am. Not. FREEEE."

And, oh the venom expressed in that declaration. I do not know the right adjectives to describe it, but his image as he voiced it is recorded indelibly in my mind. Sometime it gets in the way of good thoughts about him that I want to remember. I didn't know what to do. I called Carol. She spoke by long distance phone to him for over half an hour, and when the conversation ended he merely wept, and wept, and wept.

Daylight came. Did I go back to bed before it dawned? I don't remember.

It was our day to go to the fitness center, and we went. The technicians were good about helping him get on and off of the three pieces of exercise equipment that he still does. They set the gauge for the time limit that he works out on each piece of apparatus. When each piece had been completed, they took his pulse and recorded the required statistics on his chart.

I prepared breakfast when we got home. Should I bring the episode of the previous night up? I wasn't sure, but I did.

Sipping orange juice, I asked, "Job, do you remember anything that happened last night?"

His answer was snappish. "Some of it," he said with a hint of anger in his voice.

"What did happen?" I asked cautiously.

"You know what happened," he said rather caustically, "why should I repeat it?"

"Do you want me to leave home or stay here with you?"

"I want you to stay here with me," was his answer.

We went to a restaurant for dinner. Night came. I felt uneasy going to bed but was too tired and sleepy to stay awake. I stayed awake reading until after Job fell asleep.

January 11, 2002 (Friday)

Give the person with Alzheimer's something to do. That is the advice of the Alzheimer's Association. I have done that all along but am doubling my efforts of late trying to comply with what seems like a good suggestion.

Job vacuumed the living and dining room carpet for me then came into the bedroom and sat down. So much for trying to make him feel useful by helping with chores. I didn't push it. He has been calm all day. I carried him to the home of our friend to get his hair cut.

It is night again. He is getting undressed for bed. Soon I will go to bed also. I hope he sleeps through the night.

January 12, 2002 (Saturday)

Amy came up for a visit. It was close to 3:00 when she arrived. She always takes charge of daddy when she comes. They go together to stores, to museums, and she accompanies him on the piano while he plays his clarinet. He seems more alive, happier, when the children visit. For me, it is comforting to hear the sound of another voice, and to know that if Job becomes agitated there is someone to share my anxiety.

January 13, 2002 (Sunday)

I went to church alone. Amy and daddy stayed home. Amy wanted to cook dinner so that I could be free to rest. As usual, when it was time for her to leave for home I began to feel the sadness and sense of being all alone that always comes.

After Amy left I tried to elicit conversation from Job, but he just sat in his recliner alternating between sleeping and jerking himself about in tremors. We sat side by side for over two hours and he never once looked my way. I am afraid, never knowing what the next moment will bring.

I went downstairs to watch the evening news. He joined me and we watched TV until 9:00 before going to bed.

January 14, 2002 (Monday)

I wonder if anyone else except me lives with such a feeling of uneasiness. My nerves are shot. I live in fear because I do not know what Job's next exhibition of dementia will be.

Late this afternoon as I was trying to relax he began to pace and wander about. If I asked him a question he answered incoherently in affected throaty whispers. He sat at the kitchen table folding napkins. He does that a lot. Maybe it is something that he does at Elder Care.

He took the butter dish from the refrigerator and buttered everything in sight: napkins, paper plates, knives, forks—everything. I suggested that we go for a walk. We did, then came home and ate dinner.

I went downstairs to watch TV. He came down but was back upstairs by 7:00 and went to bed. I was so nervous. I came up to check on him and found him in bed with his shorts and a dress shirt on. I persuaded him to come with me and watch "Columbo," a TV show that we both had enjoyed once. He did watch with me, and when the show was over it was really time for bed. He slept through the night.

January 15, 2002 (Tuesday)
Job did well at the fitness center. He was even dressed appropriately, which included wearing sneakers instead of dress shoes. At home he roams about, opening and closing doors. The constant pacing is maddening. I am always afraid he will go out, but I don't say anything to him. I've taken to locking the doors a bit later at night hoping that he will feel that he has more freedom.

It is a wonderful night for sleeping. The wind is up. Our neighborhood is cemetery quiet.

When I picked Job up from Elder Care today I saw robins, lots of them. And it's only the middle of January.

January 22, 2002 (Tuesday)
The first appreciable snowfall of winter came this past Saturday. It started just as we were heading for the fitness center. In the short time we were there, the streets became treacherous.

Job shoveled part of the driveway. Later, several youngsters knocked on our door and asked if they could shovel. I was glad to pay them to do it. It is unusual for children in this neighborhood to ask to perform that task. Who can remember when shoveling snow was a well paying job for youngsters?

Job was so restless on Saturday I gave him a sedative before he went to bed. On Sunday morning he was still groggy, so we didn't go to church. I knew that he needed some kind of outing, so we went to a see a movie after dinner. By our standards the movie was poor—made to appeal to the young and immature. Before it was half over, we left and came home.

Last night I sensed that in order for me to rest I should give Job another sedative.

He was so groggy today I didn't let him exercise until after he came from Elder Care. Tonight he is unbelievably good. But oh, tomorrow, and tomorrow, and all the tomorrows to come when I must deal with this disease! I wish I could hope that things would miraculously get better. They won't, and my mind, and heart, and soul are wrenched with a dreadful suffering.

January 23, 2002 (Wednesday)
It is as I thought it would be, even though I tried to shape the course of events (it is impossible to do so) by going the extra

mile to make everything pleasant. Things went well for a while. They began to deteriorate when I went to the ATM machine located inside of the bank. We had gone on several errands. Job had complained of being cold even though the heater in the car was on. At the bank I suggested that he not get out of the car since he was already cold.

When I came back to the car he was in his trembling, shaking mode.

"What's the matter, Job?" I asked.

"It was cold inside of 'that door'," he said.

"But you didn't go inside of the bank."

His voice had risen to a loud, angry level.

"You always think I don't know what I'm talking about," he said, "I still say it was cold inside of that door that you just came out of."

I knew that I was in for trouble for the rest of the day, and I was, but with things too piddling to talk about.

It has been cloudy all day and rain has drizzled. It is night. When I put the trash to curbside I noticed how warm and like Spring it felt outside. There are absolutely no sounds in the neighborhood. I am afraid to go to sleep.

January 29, 2002 (Tuesday)

How I wish that the memory of this day could be forever erased from my mind. I would sacrifice the early part of it that had been very pleasant to have it so. I had gone to the nursery school.

It was noon when I got home from that part of my day's activities. I immediately began preparing dinner. I had put a light under a pot to cook some vegetables when the telephone rang. Answering the call, I found that it was from the nurse at Elder Care.

With profuse apologies, Jennifer, the nurse, informed me that I would have to come for Job as he had refused to be "redirected" (to or from some behavior or activity), had become very loud, and his actions were upsetting to the other clients. I told her that I would be right down, and indeed I did leave home right away.

Job was in a sorry state when I arrived at the facility. They had isolated him from the other clients. He sat in the nurse's office wrapped in a shawl that the nurse had provided. His ears, which stick way out from his head, were red, as were his eyes. He seemed angry and avoided eye contact with me and the nurse.

Jennifer spoke calmly to him in a soft voice. She touched him gently in a reassuring and caring manner. Privately, she told me that Job was in such a state of agitation that she thought he should go to the hospital. Further, she advised that it would prob-ably be best to call the police and let them transport him there. Otherwise, she feared that he would direct his hostility toward me. We checked with Dr. Miles, and he agreed that taking him to the hospital was the best course of action.

The ambulance corps arrived promptly. In my haste to get to the Elder Care facility as quickly as possible, I wasn't sure if I had turned the gas light from underneath the pot that I was using in dinner preparation, and I went home to check. When I got to the hospital Job was on a gurney in the Emergency Room.

It was early afternoon when we arrived at the hospital and very close to 8:30 at night when we left. During the entire time, Job was very agitated. He complained that he had to urinate but wasn't able to. He was given a catheter to facilitate urination and, against advice from nurses, he kept trying to dislodge it. He kept trying and finally succeeded in getting the sheet that covered the gurney totally off. Seeing that, a nurse gave him a bundle of tow-els to fold.

Perhaps it seems a battle not worthwhile fighting to get the Alzheimer's patient to wash himself and wear clean underclothes. I happen to think that is one battle that is always worth fighting even if in the final analysis you lose. Today, I lost and suffered mortal embarrassment because of it. Job had neither washed, nor put on the clean underwear that I had laid out for him, and the result of his negligence out of sheer stubbornness was very telling.

Job was eventually given medicine to bring his anxiety under control. The hospital also provided me with a few pills of the same medication to use at home if I needed to. What I wanted them to do was to keep Job in the hospital overnight. I had become very distraught and wept. Oddly, hospital staff didn't seem to understand why. I was deathly afraid to take Job home with me. When in accordance with hospital instructions we saw Dr. Miles two days later, he agreed with me that the hospital should have observed Job overnight.

January 30, 2002 (Wednesday)

I have not been outside all day. I have stayed in and administered to Job's needs. Last night when we got home from the hospital, I was surprised that he sat up until 10:45. He was still quite agitated when we got home from the hospital, so I gave him a sleeping pill and one of the pills that had been prescribed by the hospital. He got up today at 9:00. I guess he was over-medicated. When he got up, he fell. I brought a urinal and a basin of water into the bedroom and he allowed me to help him bathe. He does not need assistance in getting dressed.

Oh, how I dread the coming of night.

THIRTY-ONE

E VER SINCE THE INCIDENT OF JANUARY twenty-ninth I have been apprehensive about taking Job to Elder Care. What if he has another outburst? What if he consistently behaves adversely and the Center will not keep him as a client? What will I do with him?

It occurred to me that one remedy might be to shorten the length of hours he spends at the facility. I have done that. Still, if the telephone rings while he is there, I am always afraid to answer for fear the call is for me to come and bring him home.

February, 2002

Job has been sleeping through the night lately. If he goes to bed very early and wakes up ready to dress for daytime, I do not hesitate to give him a sleeping pill. Fearing that I might give him too many if I gave one every night, I asked our pharmacist what I should do. He suggested giving him the sedative only if he wakes up. That is working well.

Both of our children and our two grandchildren have spent time with us this month. The girls' husbands do not always come with them on visits and I understand why. I am just glad that our children are standing by me and are doing all they can to help.

While visiting, Carol called our doctor and he told her, as he has told me, that we should start "thinking of the next step" for Job. He suggested that one possibility would be to sell our home and live in an Assisted Living Community. He impressed upon us that we should not delay making plans.

His admonition not to wait until a crisis situation arose was very convincing. Procrastinating until a crisis arises, the doctor warned, could mean that Job could be placed in a facility that is not of our choosing.

Nevertheless, the advice to begin "thinking of the next step" introduced a whole new set of concerns to my already over-stressed condition. There was the idea of possibly selling my home, which would be a most unsatisfactory arrangement. How could I sell the home that is only now, except that it does not have the additional room that I wanted, is exactly how I've always wanted it to be?

Carol is still visiting. Job and I walked in our spacious back-yard to play with our soon-to-be three-year-old grandson, Julian. He wanted to play "hide-and-seek," and sometimes he, and some-times "grandpop" hid behind the large silver maple that once sup-ported a tire swing put there for his mother when she was little. Across the ditch from our yard are houses where her little play-mates lived before moving away when they, too, were little. Selling my home would mean packing up forty years of memo-ries and becoming acquainted with the unfamiliar. Still, it is an option that I may have to consider.

This month, we celebrated our forty-fifth wedding anniver-sary. The children surprised us by arranging a dinner-party for us at a very nice hotel. Most of our relatives who live in the area, as well as a few special friends, were invited to join us in the cel-ebration.

The party was on Saturday. Today, Sunday, the children have left to return to their homes. Before leaving, we all had an early dinner together. Later, in the early evening, I thought Job might be hungry again, so we went to a nearby restaurant and ate a light supper. Anticipating the loneliness that we would feel with the children gone, I decided that we would go for a drive.

When we came home from the drive, saying that he was hungry, Job headed right for the refrigerator. I made a sandwich for him and gave him a glass of milk and a piece of homemade apple pie. I had thought that going out to eat, then going for a drive would bring him some satisfaction, but no matter what I do to try to satisfy his needs, it is never enough. Amy and also a friend have told me that I must breathe in a certain way to help relieve the buildup of tension that I am experiencing. All day I have been practicing the breathing method they suggested, hoping it will ward off the stroke that I feel certain I am headed for.

March, 2002

Early in the month Dr. Miles called to see if Job has had further outbursts while at Elder Care. I was able to say that no, he has not, but that I find it best to leave him there for fewer hours. Later in the year I will find that sometimes even this doesn't work. He has not had to return to the hospital, nor has the facility called me to get him earlier than I had planned. But several times when I've arrived to bring him home he has been isolated from the group and is sitting, trembling, in the nurses' office. On these occasions it is obvious that he is experiencing agitation, as evidenced by the redness of his ears, the trembling, of course, and the fact that he will not make eye contact with anyone.

Each time we visit the doctor I ask if I should continue taking Job to exercise at the fitness center. His advice is, yes, so we continue to go for a workout three times a week. Although I have mentioned to Job that when he appears at the gym (summer, winter, spring, or fall) in a full dress suit, including a tie, he calls attention to his illness. But he continues to dress as if he is to be in the company of Heads of State. Because of this eccentricity I have had to tell everyone of Job's Alzheimer's.

Everyone is very kind and no one teases him about his always being dressed up. Some may at times remark, "Say, you're looking mighty handsome today, young man." One or two have said teasingly that all dressed up, Job makes them look slouchy in their workout suits.

We continue to engage in a few social activities, although it is becoming more and more difficult to do so. It is Friday, March 8, 2002. We went to our scheduled matinee orchestral concert. We take the commuter train downtown and usually come back to our area and eat dinner at a restaurant. While we were eating, Job grew quiet and looked despondent. I asked why and he said he didn't feel well and wanted to go home. He showed no sign of illness once we were home, but he was very restless, and although it made three consecutive nights that I had done so I gave him a sleeping pill before he went to bed.

DURING THE YEARS THAT I HAVE DEALT WITH Job's dementia-caused erratic behavior I have allowed myself to get completely out of control only several times. When I reflect on them, I wonder if even at those times I didn't just overreact to the situation, since I knew that he was not in control of his actions.

March 9, 2002 (Saturday)

We went late to the fitness center. Since Job had not felt well last night I wanted to give him as much time as he needed to get himself together before going. We came home from exercising, and I did a few chores while Job sat in the living room with his hat and jacket on.

Late in the afternoon we went to a mall. I had no shopping to do but I considered that the ride to the mall, and walking around in it for a while would help make Job tired enough to sleep through the night. I did not want to give him a sleeping pill for a fourth night.

On our way from the mall, I picked up a take-out fish dinner and we came home and ate. I suggested that we go for a walk. We left the dinner dishes and went for a very long walk around our development. He had worn dress shoes to the gym, so I asked if he wanted to change to sneakers before our walk. He chose not to change.

Immediately when we returned home he went to the closet and began changing his dress shoes for sneakers.

"Why are you doing that?" I asked.

He didn't answer but he stopped with the sneakers and began to change the shirt that he had worn all day.

"Job, why?" I asked.

"Look, I have shirts," he retorted angrily, "and if I want to change, I'll change. You just want me to do what you want me to do."

"Are you going to bed now? It's not even 6:00."

When he said yes, he was going to bed and it wasn't yet 6:00, I just lost it. After all I had done to provide enough activity to cause him to be tired enough to sleep without a sedative, he was going to bed at this unreasonable hour. I knew that he would not sleep through the night.

I cried. I screamed. I called Amy and told her (as I have told him) that I was doing all that I could do to keep him out of a nursing home, but I simply could not deal with him any longer. With the phone line still open I screamed uncontrollably. I didn't know that Amy's line was open also. When I picked my phone up to put it on the cradle she said, "Mommy, I'm coming up."

I tried to persuade her not to come all the way from Maryland, but she and her husband came anyway. She made reservations for me to stay at a hotel that is close by our home, but I wanted to stay at home, so she cancelled the reservations.

THIRTY-TWO

THE YEAR IS MOVING ALONG. With few exceptions, throughout April and May things have continued pretty much as they have for much of last year and up to the present time. It is becoming increasingly more difficult to deal with Job's behavior.

April 27, 2002 (Saturday)

At whatever time Job decides to get out of bed, I must get up too. Even if I beg him to stay in bed a while longer so that I can rest, he will not do it. Today, however, I was glad that he was up early. We had a social engagement for early afternoon, and as he was up early, we could get our fitness center obligation over with and have the afternoon free.

We had a wonderful time at the Fiftieth Wedding Anniversary celebration of our friends. I was tired from the day's activities and bought take-out food for dinner. It was after dinner that Job began to show signs of his dementia that are very distressing. He began to pack some of his clothing. He put on his jacket, and on top of that, his raincoat. He went in and out of the house. He paced, and talked, but in talking was not able to complete sentences.

Darkness was coming on. He put on my jacket and started out into the darkness.

"Job," I said to him very sternly, "if you go out of this house tonight I am going to call the police and ask them to take you somewhere, anywhere."

That, of course, made him angry. He took off the jacket and sat in a chair near the doorway.

"Let them take me to hell," he said.

"But if they do that, they will leave you here in my hell," I said, "or do you know where there is another one?"

I am agonizing now over the thought that I must "put him away some place" so that I do not have to be frightened anymore, and so that my heart can rest, and so that the tension in my upper abdomen will go away. How odious the expression "put him away" is to me. When is the right time to give up on caring for someone you love?

Admittedly, there are times when the emotion one feels for the Alzheimer's patient is not love. There are times when no matter how hard a caregiver tries, the response to some actions of the loved one being cared for is the very opposite of love. Literature from the Alzheimer's Association cautions not to take personally things the Alzheimer's patient may say or do that are hurtful. I suspect that Alzheimer's caregivers, and there are millions of them, have found it necessary to disregard this caution many times.

Hate comes as an unwelcome guest when your loved one engages in an offending behavior that seems to have been entered into deliberately. The times when I have loved Job most in his present condition are those where I have observed him trying so hard to do the right thing and still getting it all wrong. For instance, when drying the dishes for me he will open a cabinet door and look for an item (a plate or glass, etc.) like the one he is drying and will store the dried object in the right place. But it could happen that when drying silverware he would not think to look in the drawer for a like object, so all the silverware might be placed in the refrigerator, or maybe the oven.

It is always best to adhere to the Alzheimer's Association's caution and not take offenses personally, because the price of ignoring their advice exacts a heavy price in feelings of guilt that are sure to be experienced later.

Still, there are times when the situations to be dealt with require an emotion other than love. The following journal entry appears out of chronological sequence of other entries, but it provides a contrasting situation to the one where displeasure with, rather than love for, your loved one will probably prevail.

September 5, 2002 (Thursday) and September 9, 2002 (Monday)
Amy and Carol invited us to spend a day with them at the

beach. We drove to Amy's in Maryland and ate dinner with her, then rode with her to Carol's home in Virginia.

We spent a lovely day in Virginia, beginning with breakfast, which we ate sitting outside in front of a nice little restaurant. Afterwards we visited The Library of Virginia. It is a very large library that Carol wanted us to visit and see the exhibit of a Blues singer who is Job's distant relative.

Saturday was spent at Virginia Beach. Job and I sunned on the beach while Amy helped Carol keep up with Julian and Alana, who always headed for the water. We did not stay over night at the beach. On Sunday we spent the morning at Carol's before heading back to Maryland where we spent the night with Amy and James.

Our drive back to Pennsylvania on Monday morning was very pleasant. I made good time driving and it was still within the range of breakfast time when we arrived at home. Rather than go out to eat, I decided to prepare breakfast at home. I discovered the calamity that would set the tone for the rest of the day when I went to the freezer in the basement to bring up a container of frozen orange juice.

The lights did not come on when I turned on the switch. I felt that a fuse (I didn't realize that we had circuit breakers rather than fuses) had blown, but I would get the juice and later ask my neighbor to do whatever was necessary to get the lights back on. As I was getting the juice I discovered puddles of water from both freezers all over the floor, and to my horror found that both freezers had defrosted, leaving many packages of vegetables, and several kinds of meat, fish, and poultry thawing.

My neighbor came over to help me. When he tripped the circuit breaker, a large flame blazed underneath the smaller freezer and we quickly disconnected it. Dwayne, my neighbor, suggested that I call the Electric Company. I did, but was told that I should call an electrician, as the problem did not come under the purview of the Electric Company's responsibility.

Within minutes after he examined the faulty freezer, the electrician found the cause of the problem. The generator of the smaller freezer had burned out. Even if I could remember the other technicalities that he pointed out, only one is important. He said the generator had been building up to the burnout level for years! And that we were lucky to have come home to a house still standing rather than one burned down to a pile of ashes!

Maybe I continued to prepare breakfast. I don't remember. What I do remember is that I began to cook the meat and poultry that had not completely thawed so that I could refreeze it. Fish and processed meats were thrown away. Vegetables were left in tact. I had to mop up the water from both defrosted freezers, even though one would be disposed of. Water from the floor was mopped up.

By dinnertime I had been going non-stop for the entire day. Still, I prepared a very good dinner, which we ate at our usual time, 5:30. With dinner over, and the kitchen cleaned up, I sat down to watch the hour of news aired on the Public Broadcasting Station. Later I went down to the rec room to watch "Columbo."

The program had just begun when I heard Job doing things in the kitchen. I called for him to come down and watch with me. When he didn't come down I came up to the kitchen to investigate what he was doing.

"What are you doing?" I asked. "Why don't you come down and watch with me?"

"I'm getting ready to eat," he said. He had food and dishes out.

"But you just ate," I said.

"Yeah, yeah," he said. He got loud and accused me of always finding fault with everything he did.

"It's you who don't do things right. You don't care anything about me. If you did," he said, "things would be better."

Could I in this moment have loved him? This would be the last time that I completely lost control. I cried. I screamed. I picked up the phone to call Carol but put it down before completing the call. Oh, God, Oh, God, Oh, GOD, I prayed, what am I to do?

May, 2002

Lawnmowers in our development started humming in late March and early April as neighbors began mowing their lawns. Now they are in full swing. The usual flowers are blooming but I only see them when I hang Job's T-shirts and my towels on the clothesline outside. To conserve what little energy I have, I no longer hang my full wash outside. I do not have (and have never wanted) a dryer. Laundry that dries more quickly I hang on lines in our full basement.

Job continues to act irrationally, with irrational behavior becoming more frequent and more intense. Sometimes he puts on layers of clothing, sometimes he packs clothing in bags or boxes, and sometimes he just takes all of his slacks and suits from the closet and lays them on a chair in the living room. Occasionally he puts a bundle of them in the car. I do not try to dissuade him from doing these things. I merely put them away when he goes to bed.

More and more he talks "off subject." That is to say, in conversation his responses are not likely to be apropos to the topic under discussion. He will never engage in any task that I suggest, but sometimes on his own initiative will pull a few weeds from a flowerbed or pick up fallen twigs.

We attend less often now the Lutheran church where Job has attended and been active in the forty years we've lived in our present community. We now prefer the African Methodist Episcopal Church service that we are more familiar with. Occasionally we go to the AME church in Ardmore, the western suburb where Job grew up, and where I met him.

Keeping his membership in that church was not practical, the travel distance being prohibitive. But we have often visited just to keep in touch with family and friends who still worship there. Job did the driving whenever we went to Ardmore. We would take the Turnpike to the Blue Route, take that to the St. Davids exit, and take Pennsylvania Route 30 east through Villanova, Rosemont, Bryn Mawr, and on into Ardmore.

As we passed through all the little towns, Job would point out familiar places: Bryn Mawr hospital where our son was born, the playground where he played as a boy, McConaghy's Funeral parlor, the railroad station, and lots of other places. As years went by he pointed out buildings (and shopping centers!) that were new to the area since he lived there.

Now I must do the driving. I am familiar with the main routes to take but have always relied on Job to tell me exactly which streets to use to get to the church. Sadly, Job is no longer able to give me directions. Recently we attended a funeral at the church and had to ask directions several times before finding the right location of the church.

May 20, 2002 (Monday)
    I feel very sad today. Maybe it is because of the letdown after yesterday's high when I attended my fifty-fifth High School class reunion. Probably the thing that has me on the verge of tears is Job's downcast look of depression. I have told him how his depressed countenance affects me.
    "Job," I've said, " why do you look so depressed? Seeing you like that makes ME unhappy. Is there anything I can do to help? Is there anything that you want to do?"
    "I don't know what to do with myself," he answered without changing his expression, and added, "but I don't want to make you unhappy.

JOB CONTINUES TO BE MOUSE QUIET all day every day. More and more he gets confused completing simple tasks. Often he changes outfits several times a day. It seems that at least one of the changes is made when I am in a hurry to get to some place. I do realize that his increasingly irrational behavior is a signal that the dementia is becoming more than I, without sacrificing my own health, can continue to cope with. My head acknowledges that it is time for him to be in a different setting; my heart does not.
    I have told our children of the doctor's warning that we should not procrastinate in making the decisions that we will surely have to make in the not too distant future. Although in miles she is not close to the situation, emotionally Carol is, and she has voiced her opinion that she is not ready for daddy to go to a nursing home. Neither am I, but something must be done before I go insane.
    The thing that makes it so difficult to come to a decision to write him off as someone who can no longer be cared for at home is that some days, or at least part of some days, he appears to be almost his old self.
    His personality is most likely to imitate pre Alzheimer's Job early in the morning, but the good-personality/bad-personality can alternate not only from day to day, but from hour to hour, and even from moment to moment. When he has good moments,

times when he is willing to be "redirected" to a more desirable behavior, I comment about it, telling him how wonderful it is that he is behaving in such a good way.

Thus it may happen that during the day I say to myself, 'things are bad but not so bad that I cannot deal with them'. But by nightfall, when he insists that he has to go to work, or to the hospital, or he thinks that he is to go somewhere but isn't sure where, I say to myself, 'this is it. I cannot stand this any longer'. It is particularly troubling when he refuses to go to bed at night, or when he awakens in the wee hours of the morning and insists on staying up. There have been nights when he did not go to bed the entire night.

May 30, 2002 (Thursday)

I had a hairdresser appointment today, so I left Job at Elder Care. I was glad that I was finished with that appointment early so that Job would not have to stay long at Elder Care. When I stopped to pick him up he was sitting apart from the group trembling and with his head bowed down. The nurse said he had not been a problem but had told her that he wanted to be by himself. He had refused to eat lunch.

Once we were home, I prepared a good lunch for him and for a while I felt that he was coming out of his depression, but he didn't.

It may be that I actually heard, either on the classical music station that our kitchen radio is always tuned to, or as a public service announcement on television, that prolonged periods of depression can be detrimental to a person's physical well-being.

By whatever means it came into my consciousness, I decided that Job's continued state of depression should be called to the attention of one of his doctors. I opted for the neurologist.

May 31, 2002 (Friday)

Job was up very early. I prepared his breakfast while still in my robe and slippers. Just as I was preparing my bath, he announced that he was going for a walk.

"No, Job," I said, "not until I finish my bath."

Surprisingly, he was compliant. When he went for a walk later, I sat in the car and watched him walk a ways up our street then turn around and head for home.

I've called a friend and inquired about nursing homes.

He still is in a state of depression that is thick and dark, and can best be described as resembling dark clouds announcing an impending storm.

Dr. Howard was not at all surprised when I told him about the depression. Although his office would be closed before I could drive down to it, he left a prescription so that I could get the anti-depressant medication without waiting until Monday when his office would be open again.

June 1, 2002 (Saturday)

Just for an outing, we went to a shopping mall. Macy's had men's suits on sale, so I bought one that Job liked. He also bought several pairs of summer slacks and some new neckties. He seemed very happy to be getting new things. We ate lunch at "Friday's." By the time we got home it was late afternoon. As soon as we got home Job did what he has done consistently for the past few weeks. He promptly sat in a chair with his hands folded between his legs and with his head bowed down looking darkly depressed.

"Oh, Job," I asked him, "do you have any idea how your looking depressed affects me?" He made no answer.

"Am I the cause of your downward look?" I asked him.

"I don't know," he replied.

"Is it the house that makes you sad? You seem fine when we are out."

"It has nothing to do with you or the house," he said.

"Do you want to live in this house or do you want me to put you in an assisted living facility?" I asked him.

"I want to live here with you," was his answer.

"What do you want to do?" I asked.

"I like going to stores. I like going to movies."

"But you must understand, Job, that I simply cannot spend all of my time going to stores and to movies."

THIRTY-THREE

ON AN ALZHEIMER'S ASSOCIATION FLYER that I have received, there is a list of behaviors that a caregiver may expect to see in a person with "dementing illness". Eleven traits are listed. They include rapidly changing mood, weeping, blushing, anger, agitation, violent striking out, stubbornness, anxiety, pacing, paranoia, and wandering.

With Job's dementia I have experienced all but two included in the listing. They are, (1) violent striking out, and (2) paranoia. Job has never been physically combative with me or with anyone else. That is not to say that at some point further along in the illness he will not do so. He has also shown no sign of paranoia with me, although the Director at Elder Care reported that Job had accused members of her staff of trying to "take his money." I feel very positive that no one had tried to do that.

The same flyer suggests some causes that may trigger certain behaviors and approaches that may be helpful in dealing with them. I will not list their suggestions from either category. However, I hope it is permissible to use their wording to express what I have experienced to be true for me, since whatever wording I would use would not convey a different message:

"What works today may not work tomorrow. It may work for someone else and not for you today; tomorrow may be different. There are no rights or wrongs in this business (of caring for an Alzheimer's patient). If your efforts cause a catastrophic reaction, it doesn't mean that you did something wrong, it means it didn't work today."

June 3, 2002 (Monday)

Today I went alone to visit one of several Assisted Living facilities that our doctor has suggested I might want to consider for Job.

June 5, 2002 (Wednesday)

If there were someone who would be a companion for Job for a few hours a day it would provide some respite for me. Today I interviewed a man whose name was on a list provided by the County as someone willing to do that work. From the moment he arrived at our home I had a feeling he would not accept the job offer. He promised that he would call and let me know of his decision, but no call ever came.

I have called an agency and enlisted the help of home health care aids to help with Job's care. They will work any eight-hour shift of my choosing. I have chosen an overnight shift so that I can sleep through the night. They will also do light housekeeping chores for me. With help, during the day I feel a little less tired, but no less anxious about things in general.

Sometimes at night when Job is very restless I get out of bed and sit in his recliner and sleep. Sometimes, after I have given him a sedative I make a pallet at the foot of the bed and sleep. It is more comfortable than the recliner. Also, I can hear him if he tries to get up. I need to hear him so that if he is too groggy from the sedative, I can help him get into the bathroom without falling if he gets up to go.

June 14, 2002 (Friday)

We used our ticket for the final orchestra concert of the season today. For the past year I have looked for a really nice restaurant where we could have lunch within the hour that we have to kill between our arrival downtown and the time the concert starts. When attending our last concert I discovered such a place, a nice Italian bistro.

That is where I planned to have dinner after today's concert, but Job wanted to come home.

We take the regional train downtown and leave our car on the large parking lot at the train station when we attend concerts. Job tried to help me locate the car when we got back to the station. He spotted one that did look similar to ours, but a lady was in it.

"Is that our car?" he asked. "Isn't that Myrna (me) in it?"

When we reached home and were getting out of the car he took all of the things that are always left in the glove compartment out of it.

In my very sweetest voice I said, "Oh, you don't need to take those out."

"And why can't we take our clothes in our own house, huh?" he said rather belligerently.

"It's just that those are items I usually leave in the car," I said in a non-criticizing way.

He continued to enter the house carrying the ice scraper, cloth for wiping the windows, pencils, directions to Carol and Amy's homes, and sundries. I did not pursue the matter further. No one knows what I am going through. Absolutely no one knows the myriad little annoyances that occur in my daily life to make it intolerable.

June 17, 2002 (Monday)

Carol came for a visit today. She is going with me to visit Assisted Living facilities.

June 19, 2002 (Wednesday)

We visited one assisted living facility yesterday and two today. When we were ready to leave the one we visited yesterday, Job said, "Well, I'll see you later." He thought we had gotten him a room at that facility. Maybe he is ready for a change even if I am not.

Of the two that we saw today, both Carol and I like one of them, and she is urging me to send in the required holding deposit.

June 22 through 25, 2002 (Saturday, Sunday, Monday, Tuesday)

Alexandra, my great-niece, lives in upstate New York and will graduate from high school on Monday night. Amy and James are coming up and they, Carol and her children are going to drive to New York for the graduation. Aunt Lois came up from the city and will ride with them. Job will go also. I had planned to attend the graduation but I am so tired and nervous I just want to stay at home and rest and unwind. Maybe the knot in my stomach will go away.

They left for New York on Saturday. On Sunday I did not attend church. I ate breakfast out and spent the rest of the day relaxing. I went to Rita's in Huntingdon Valley and bought a water ice. I didn't cook dinner, just ate leftovers already in the refrigerator. In the evening, Steven, my nephew and Alexandra's father called and said his Uncle Job had had a good day, was lively, and interacted well with everyone. Maybe there is hope that it will be a long time before he needs to go into a facility.

Today, Monday, I did only things that I wanted to do. Towards evening I began to tense up again, contemplating that tomorrow Job will come home. I've missed him but still dread the thought of having to deal with his mood swings, his stubbornness, his agitation, his pacing, and packing, and all the other eccentricities peculiar to his dementia.

I do not want to put him in a facility until it is absolutely necessary. When will that be? Should I make it soon? Should I wait? Only I can make the decision. I lie awake at night pondering the answer, while my heart thumps so heavily in my chest it feels as if it is turning over, and while inside my head an inaudible screaming is taking place.

The screams are piercing, and are reminiscent of those I uttered when I was in labor with my firstborn child. A small amount of some anesthesia—gas, I believe—was administered as pangs from contractions occurred. For a time during the birthing process I endured the sharp contractions with reserved groans of agony. But when the time for bearing down and pushing came, I remember uttering what seemed to me to be one long, continuous series of screams, as the pain became unbearable.

They came home today, Tuesday. Job seemed very tired. He slept through the night.

July 5, 2002 (Friday)

Job got out of bed very early, but it was 6:00 by the time he bathed, dressed, and came out to breakfast, which I prepared. My intention was to take him to Elder Care for a few hours, although this is not his usual day for going.

I was busy in another part of the house when I heard him continue to pray after he had said his table grace. When I didn't hear him anymore I sat down to the table with him and we talked. He began to weep silently and said through his tears that he tries to "do the right thing."

He seems to be slipping farther and farther into darkness of mind, and he seems to realize that that is happening to him.

It is a beautiful morning. The heat and humidity of yesterday are gone. After he finished his breakfast, I suggested that we sit in the yard for a while. We did. Yesterday, trying to find a cool place to escape the intense heat, we had moved a table from the patio and placed it in the shade of the silver maple tree that sets in the center of the back lawn. Today we sat under the tree and observed daylilies growing in a clump near the ditch. Job had removed the flowers and placed them where they would not be destroyed while work was being done to the ditch. Some, he didn't have time to remove before the Township workmen came to do their work. Those that remained are blooming in elegant splendor along the two-hundred-foot-long bank of the ditch.

We sat for a long time just enjoying the out-of-doors. Presently I went to the shed and got gardening tools and we took turns cultivating around our twelve tomato plants.

July 20 (Saturday) through July 25, 2002 (Thursday)

The children are doing an excellent job of helping me care for their father. He is going to spend a week with Carol. Amy came to our house to take him to Virginia in her car to Carol and Aaron's home. He should enjoy our grandchildren. I've written detailed instructions for Carol so that she will know what to expect and what to do in order to make daddy's visit with her as enjoyable as possible for him, and as carefree for herself as possible.

Without having to care for Job I have relaxed, gone to exercise on our regularly scheduled days, I have not cooked three meals a day, and I have had no trouble sleeping. In a few hours, that will change. James has called and said they will arrive here in a few hours bringing Job home from his visit with Carol. Already I can feel the muscles in my stomach tightening, and a tears-producing lump forming in my throat.

Until they arrive, I will sit on the patio listening to cicadas singing in the round.

August, 2002

There is no quality of life for either Job or me. We exist together. Still, I am loath to let him go. Even with help coming in at night, things are difficult for me. During the huge chunk of daylight hours after the home health care aides have left and I become the sole caregiver, I must constantly be on duty chauffeuring him from place to place to keep him entertained.

Also, I must interrupt whatever task I am engaged in to check on his whereabouts to see that he hasn't wandered away. Often he will slip quietly out of the house and when I check, he is pulling weeds from a flowerbed or picking up fallen twigs. I may check several times and he is occupied with that work. But the next time I look, he may have taken off down the street. I do not let many minutes pass without checking to see if he is still on our grounds.

August 16, 2002 (Friday)

Carol and her children have visited with us for a couple of days. I remarked to her that sometimes daddy seems unaffected by dementia. She said she knows.

We spent most of today getting her to the train station so that they could return to their home in Virginia. It was after 3:00 when we got home. We had no sooner entered the house than Job sat down, retied his shoelaces for the umpteenth time, and announced, "Well, I'm ready."

"Ready for what?" I screamed.

"I don't know," he said, "I thought you said we were going somewhere."

At night, he went to bed without incident, no refusing to get undressed, no refusing to put on pajamas, and as he got into bed he said, "I still love you."

The words sounded very sincere, just as they always have.

I have tried to remedy the problem of always being Job's constant caregiver by having an around the clock home health aide. That has not worked out well. If anything, it has added to my anxiety and frustration. It is not easy having a total stranger adjust to your established routine. Now, I am back to having an aide only from late night until early morning, even though I have observed for many weeks that Job sleeps through the night. No matter how quietly I go about the house, shortly after the home health care aide leaves, I find Job up and making up the bed.

September, 2002

This month is bringing with it new concerns. One activity I have counted on to fill up a few hours of the day has been to go by train to the city. Recently I discovered that even this is no longer a pleasurable option.

Job's electric razor needed repairing (again) and I knew of a shop in the city that could do the repair. I planned to go into the city by train, get the razor repaired, and find a nice place to eat lunch before coming home. There are thirteen train stops between our boarding station and the station where we would get off. We had not gone past more than five of them before Job wanted to know when we would get off the train.

"Not for a while yet," I reassured him.

"Oh," he said, "they've changed the stations around, then."

"No," I said, "the stations are right where they were when you passed by them commuting to work for twenty-five years."

He wasn't convinced, and when the conductor came to collect tickets he actually grabbed him by the arm and questioned him about the right station for us to get off the train. I managed to get the conductor's eye and signaled that all was not well with Job. He understood immediately and was very patient and reassuring.

"Where're you going, Buddy," he asked Job. I supplied the answer.

"You're not there yet," the conductor said, continuing, "I tell you what I'll do. I'll call out your station when we get to it, okay?"

After that, Job relaxed. On the return trip home he got up several times to get off the train. Luckily, unlike previous rides, I had not fallen asleep and intercepted before he got off at a wrong station.

October, 2002

The screaming inside my head is constant as Job's dementia progresses toward a more severe stage. I know from Alzheimer's Association flyers (and from consultations with the neurologist and our family doctor) that even in the severe stage a patient can live for a long time. I'm not certain that Job has reached that stage. I do not know all of the conditions that the severe stage of the disease entails.

It is my understanding that Alzheimer's dementia may reduce the sufferer to complete helplessness and they become unable to feed or bathe themselves, and are unable to control all bodily functions. Job is not yet a victim of any of these infirmities, but his recent behavior makes it more difficult for me to deal with him.

Every night, usually after supper, he insists that he must go to work. Even earlier in the day he will put on hat and jacket (he always puts on a hat and jacket, sometimes two jackets, sometimes three) and announce that he is going somewhere. He may do this several times during the day.

The cursing and accusations that "I don't give a damn about him" I can endure. But during these times of his wanting to get out, I unlock the doors so he can go, because I do not want him to become so agitated that I must take him to the hospital to be calmed down. Of course, if he does go out, I get in the car and follow him. I do not offer to take him into the car with me. I merely follow him until he is again safely in our driveway.

THIRTY-FOUR

So many negative things have happened over the past month, there is no doubt in my mind that what happened next was providential.

In July I sent the "holding deposit" to the assisted living facility that we had decided on for Job. At that time I asked if they could hold the check until such time as I felt that Job needed to move into their facility. I wanted assurance that if a room became available sooner than I felt Job needed to move into it, they would release the space to someone else but continue to hold my deposit until I needed it. It was a delaying tactic on my part. I wanted to, and felt that I could, care for Job at home for as long as it was possible for me to do so.

I was assured that this arrangement was possible, but as it turned out, it was not a possibility at all. I remember how relaxed I had felt in July after sending in the deposit. I had after all done what the doctor said I should do, placed my name on a list of a place where Job could go in case a crisis situation arose whereby he could no longer be cared for at home.

My old anxieties returned when I got a call from the marketing director of the facility telling me that if I did not anticipate an immediate move in, they would have to return my deposit. A few days later the check came by mail. By now our children realized that they would have to intervene to help me do what they (and our doctor) knew to be the wise and right thing to do.

"Mom, you're getting sick," Carol remarked. "We're losing daddy. We don't want to lose you as well."

Both girls, Carol and Amy, worked together filling out papers, consulting with Dr. Miles, consulting with the assisted living facility, and handling all other transactions relating to their father's move from the place that had been home to him for forty years and three months. I was so overwrought, and so mentally and emotionally exhausted at having to make such a profound decision that I hadn't the physical endurance to undertake the tasks they willingly, and lovingly, performed for me.

The one thing that neither of our children could do was to sign the check to pay the facility. That ignoble deed was left for me alone to accomplish. Job accompanied me to the bank. The day was damp and bleak. A "nor'easter," forecast for today on the previous evening's news, had indeed come to pass. Rain, cold and chilling, fell intermittently throughout the day.

Carol had given me the date, which was the date of this rainy day, that she had promised the director of the facility that I would have the check to her. Hoping to delay delivering the check for as long as possible, I called Carol and said that since it was raining so hard I thought I would wait another day before handing in the check.

"Mommy, take her the check," Carol said, firmly, but not in an unkind tone of voice.

"Take her the check. She's waiting for it," Carol said again.

I agreed to do so, and Job and I drove to the facility together and delivered it.

From the time I awoke in the morning, I had spells of weeping, knowing of the thing that I must do. On the way to the bank, I wept, but Job didn't notice. This was not unusual. We would ride for hours in the car together and his eyes would never even glance casually in my direction.

On leaving the bank, I wept, and in the car on the way home, tears continued to flow. I held Job's hand, and, through wracking sobs, tried to impart to him what was about to happen in our lives.

"Job," I said, "I must tell you something."

"What?" he wanted to know.

"We are not going to be able to live together any longer," I said.

"But why?" He asked.

"Because you are sick and I can't take care of you anymore."

"Well, I don't feel sick," he said.

"I know, but you are," I told him.

"Why are you crying?" he asked, as if we had had no con-versation at all about the matter.

"Oh, Job, Job, Job," I cried, "I'm crying because I love you, and because you are sick, and because we must now live in sep-arate places."

Out of this traumatic experience that has intruded itself into my life, I've learned something about tears that I never imagined before. I now conceptualize them, not as mere drops of salty liq-uid, but as entities governed by a guiding influence instructing them on when to become activated. How many times during the course of Job's illness have I longed for tears to break through the barrier set up by the constrictive lump in my throat and flow? That at least would have expressed the sadness that was within my heart. But they would not come.

By what means could my tears have known to expend them-selves in such niggardly quantities over these past four years when I wanted them to come at my bidding? It is as if they had the wisdom to hold back and build up the reservoir required for me to get through this stressful time when there seems to be no end to the buckets full that are needed.

The move-in was scheduled for October twentieth, Sunday. On Saturday we went to the facility and prepared the room that Job would occupy with some of his familiar belongings. We car-ried up his clothing, bed sheets, a comforter, and family pictures. Carol had framed a very nice picture of Alana and Julian that had been taken in a lovely garden setting. This she hung over the head of his bed. The several plaques he had received from the Township for dedicated service as a Library Board member were mounted neatly on the wall.

Amy had bought a small CD and tape player. From his volu-minous collection of CD's of classical music, she selected five or six that she knew he would enjoy listening to. More will be car-ried up later. He will not know how to operate the CD player but perhaps someone will be available to help him.

And now, the day is upon us. Oh, God, how can I stand it? We decided to do it this way: Carol, Amy, and Julian would take Job to the facility and have lunch with him. Aaron kept Alana at home because she is too little to be expected to behave well eating out. The children would come back to the home of their childhood, then leave for their present homes. I would go to the facility at 5:00 and eat dinner with Job, then I would come home to an empty house.

The children, with Job, were not out of our driveway on their way to the facility before I became overcome with involuntary emotion. Tactfully, Aaron went with little Alana to the rec room to watch cartoons. On this overcast but still middle-of October warm day, the two of them later walked about in our backyard. Through a haze of tears, I kept busy with inconsequential household chores. To try and focus my thought on something other than the awful truth facing me, I went to several stores. Nothing helped.

By late afternoon, minus Job, the children came home with nothing on their countenance to suggest that parting with their father had been a tearful one (although probably not in his presence). I would not have known of that occurrence had not a gentleman, a resident of the facility, unintentionally informed me.

The gentleman informant and Job were sitting at the table together when I joined them for dinner.

In a heavy Bavarian accent he inquired if Job were my father.

"Oh, no," I laughingly responded, "Job is my husband."

"Ah," he apologized profusely, "my eyesight is not so good that I could make that distinction."

"That's OK," I said. "Neither of us is offended. He knows that he is only a year and a half older than I am. My hair is not all white like his because I wouldn't let him worry me to death all these years that we've been married."

"So you are his wife," he declared more than questioned. "Then they were your children who were so upset earlier?"

"They were our children. Were they upset?"

"Oh, yes, very," he said with a proper degree of sobriety.

Pondering the deceptive façade that the children presented when they came home evoked emotions of grief that, miraculously, I was able to suppress.

AT THIS WRITING, THREE WEEKS HAVE PASSED since that fateful day. During his first week in the facility, I visited Job twice a day, once at breakfast time, and again either during the lunch or supper hour. Before leaving I would encourage him to walk with me to his room, away from the in-house "Courtyard", where residents in various degrees of physical and mental deterioration congregated.

In the room we would stand in a full body embrace as we did long ago, my arms around him, his around me. Then, such a posture sent electrical charges of passion through our bodies. Now, there is no passion, only a deep and abiding caring. For the first time in almost three years, since his dementia caused his personality to change so profoundly, I am free to just love him. The barrier that stood between my ability to love him completely— intolerable behavior, including verbal abuse—is absorbed by facility caregivers.

He appears very frail. Almost nothing that he says shows any connection to the real world, but he still knows his name, and mine. Every time I visit I ask him, "Who am I?" He smiles and says, "You're Myrna." And the sound of that is sweet to me.

I HAD MY OWN PREVIOUSLY SCHEDULED physical checkup recently. Mostly, the doctor was concerned with my emotional wellbeing.

"You did the right thing, Mrs. Winters."

"Yes. Hearing you say it, I am reassured."

"How is he doing?"

"He seems to be adjusting. I visit him every day."

"I'd like you to not visit everyday. You need to get away. Go to lunch with a friend. Take a vacation."

"But if I don't visit he might forget me."

"He is going to forget you anyway. Set out a picture of yourself where he can see it."

"All right."

"Do you need medication to help you get through this?"

"No. I am going to try to manage without it."

Dr. Miles has been wonderful to both Job and me through this and other illnesses, so I want to follow his advice now. But to ask me not to visit Job every day, to hold his hand, to reassure him that the children and I love him, is more than I can presently contemplate. It is almost as if I have been asked to mop the Atlantic Ocean dry using only paper towels to do the job. Still, I know that for my own welfare, I must follow the doctor's orders.

November 11, 2002 (Monday)
I talked to Carol today. I told her how I learned about how difficult it was for them to leave daddy at the facility on the Sunday that they carried him there.

"How did you find out?" she asked.

"A little birdie told me," I said.

"Amy didn't cry. Julian wanted to know why I was crying," she said. "I wasn't going to tell you this because I knew it would upset you. On our way home Julian told his dad that I said 'we have to get daddy out of that place.'"

"Don't you still think we should?" I asked.

"No, mommy, no. We shouldn't." She said.

So AMY DIDN'T SHED TEARS. I know that it was not because she didn't feel sadness about what has transpired.

Always the quiet, sensitive, serious daughter, Amy, in her adult years, has learned to change things if she can, but to accept graciously those that she can not.

MY BIRTHDAY WAS IN SEPTEMBER. Job has always insisted on selecting the card that he wants to give to the children or to me. I could never buy a birthday card that read, "From both of us," because he wanted the card to reflect his sentiments. And he would always write a little note at the bottom of the card.

Over the years, cards we bought for each other would be left in various places for the other to find. Sometimes he would leave mine on his dresser, and sometimes it would be left at my place at the table. I would do the same with cards I bought for him.

I knew that he would not remember the date of my birthday, so the day before my special day, I carried the home health aide with us to the drug store so that Job could buy a birthday card for me.

"Here's money to pay for the card," I told the aide. "You walk away from him and let him make his card selection, then you pay the cashier."

She walked away and he spent a long time choosing his card. From another part of the store I watched him pick up one card after another, read it and replace it in the rack. Finally he found one that satisfied him. At home he placed the card in the envelope and left it in his jewelry box

I knew that he would not remember to give me the card, so on the morning of my birthday, I took the card from the jewelry box to read it.

On the first page, written in large type were the words"

My Wife—

Underneath that in smaller, capitalized print it read:

*MY VERY
BEST FRIEND*

A picture of a bouquet of roses in a delicately decorated cup and saucer separated the above words from these in smaller print:

*Because I feel so good about myself
When I'm with you
Because I trust and count on you
To help me see things through...*

The verse continues on the first page of the inside fold:

*Because
You understand
My moods
And accept me
At my worst,
Because you try
To give support
And put my feelings
First...*

The verse concludes on the second page of the inside fold:

*Because of how you share and live,
I give you all I have to give,
With love for all you are to me—*

And everything you've helped me be.

Happy Birthday
Happiness Forever

The card was not signed. I wrote on it: From Job, 2002. He picked it out himself.

IT IS LONELY BEING A WIDOW OF ANY KIND, I suppose. An Alzheimer's widow certainly has a very lonely life. Job is still living and breathing, I still carry him to keep doctor's appointments, but he no longer sleeps beside me, or accompanies me to the grocery store, and I must push the grocery cart myself.

Yes, living with him became difficult. Yes, my health was suffering because of constantly caring for him. But because he never became physically "combative" with me I think I shall always wonder if by sending him away I betrayed the trust in me that he had.

EPILOGUE

NOT QUITE THREE MONTHS HAVE PASSED since Job was accepted and went to live in an assisted living facility that adver-
tised in the Alzheimer's section of AN AREA GUIDE TO
SENIOR RESIDENCES AND CARE OPTIONS. He was a good
candidate to be in such a facility. He was ambulatory, continent,
and able to shower (I did request in writing that he be given
assistance in bathing) and dress himself. Our primary care physician completed the forms that the facility required of him.

Satisfied that the right action had been taken to avoid having
to make a hasty move in the event a "crisis" situation arose, at
night I slept peacefully. During the day I completed necessary
tasks and even engaged in a few activities just because they were
fun and relaxing.

And every day I visited Job. Sometimes we went for a drive
to the mall. Other times we would stop for ice cream at a restaurant that specialized in that treat. On Sundays we went to church.
On the advice of our doctor that it was all right to do so, we
continued to go to the fitness center three times a week to exercise. I carried Job to keep doctor's appointments that had already
been scheduled. We even attended an orchestral concert performed by our local symphony orchestra. On none of these out-
ings did I ever bring him back to our home.

AN INTERLUDE JUST SHORT OF TWO MONTHS HAS PASSED. I have discovered that the nightmare I thought had been avoided by placing Job in a facility to deal with Alzheimer's dementia has only
just begun.

After October, 2002, I became lax in making daily journal

entries, so I have no accurate dates of when the circumstances began that have caused me presently to experience a higher level of stress than I did during the total time I dealt with Job's illness.

IN NOVEMBER, JUST ONE MONTH INTO HIS STAY at the Facility I visited Job during the supper hour. All was well when I left for home, but shortly after I arrived a call came that my husband was being sent to our local hospital because of an attempted physical episode with another resident. Job's behavior was described to me as being very agitated. Nevertheless, the hospital did not keep him for an overnight stay for observation as the facility had hoped. When I saw him the next day he was very heavily sedated.

On my visit the next day, Sunday, he was so sedated that during the three hours or more of my visit, he did not wake up.

During the next week my husband was seen at the facility by their psychiatrist. I spoke with the psychiatrist, stating that although Job had not shown aggressive behavior when I cared for him I understood that the potential for it was one of the properties of the dementia.

By week's end I received a call that because of my husband's aggressive, combative behavior he was being sent to what I would learn later was a psychiatric hospital. He would be kept there for from five to seven days to be "evaluated."

"What will you do to correct the undesirable behavior?" I asked the attending psychiatrist.

"We will keep him until his condition is 'stabilized'." Those are the nearest words I can remember of the psychiatrist's reply.

"Then what will happen to him?" I asked.

"After he's stabilized we'll send him back to the facility."

WHILE HE WAS IN THAT HOSPITAL JOB COMPLAINED of chest pains and was sent to a medical hospital close by the asylum that he was in. After a two-day stay at the medical hospital he was discharged and returned to where his aggressive behavior was being "evaluated."

My experience with Job was that once a property of the Alzheimer's condition presented, it did not go away. When I was caring for him and noticed that agitation had become a constant component of his demeanor I told our primary care physician and he prescribed something to combat the condition. Likewise, when I called Job's depression to the attention of the neurologist, he prescribed medication to alleviate it. I understood clearly that once begun, however undesirable, the new conditions would not go away but could be controlled with medication.

I was nervously suspicious that the remedy for this present behavior would be a drug that would make Job constantly lethargic. I reasoned, in other words, that the combative behavior would necessarily need to be controlled by drugs stronger than the ones he was already taking, and I have mentioned the consequence of unacceptable sluggishness they produced.

I visited Job in both hospitals. He appeared very ill in the medical hospital but the doctor's found no abnormality in the functioning of his heart. In the psychiatric hospital he was fairly clear-headed and responded positively to my presence. Hospital staff told me that he had on other occasions been combative and on the day of my last visit was extremely agitated after I left the premises.

More and more the thought uppermost in my mind was that once Job was returned to the original facility the combativeness would continue. The psychiatrist assured me, however, that once Job was "stabilized" he would be ready to return. I assumed that even if there were still some combativeness the facility would know how to handle it since they had accepted Job as a resident knowing that he had been diagnosed to have Alzheimer's dementia.

Job remained in the psychiatric hospital for several more days. The call came that he would be returning to the facility. The stress that I was experiencing had become overwhelming. A number of concerns caused the stress. Among them were Job's unexpected visits to hospitals, the facility calling to tell me of new development's in his behavior. They called and requested that I order (I was purchasing Job's medications from the VA) medicines they had asked our doctor to prescribe for him. They called to say that Job was to be seen by a psychiatrist. The psychiatrist consulted with me about what might be better insurance arrangements to handle costs that might be incurred in treating Job's illness.

This new level of stress had so overwhelmed me that I had to ask my children to help. I asked the facility to direct all phone calls relating to anything regarding Job to my oldest daughter Carol.

So, although it was I who received the call from the social worker at the psychiatric hospital informing me that Job would be returning to the facility, it was the facility manager and Carol who discussed the conditions of his return.

Because of his combative behavior, Job could no longer be a resident at that facility.

"How could this be?" I wondered. "Hadn't the psychiatrist certified that Job was 'stabilized?'"

We questioned the psychiatrist about it. He said that apparently after he had made his determination that Job was stabilized, Job had other incidents of combativeness that were not called to his attention.

The facility administrator informed Carol that Job could remain at the facility only until we could find another place for him. In the meantime, we would have to pay someone (in addition to continuing to pay the facility) to be one-on-one with him at all times.

On the very first night of his return to the facility Job became so agitated that I was called to come to the facility and "quiet him down." I couldn't believe that this was happening, that I was being asked to come and perform a function that I was paying a large sum of money for the facility to perform.

I know the words to use, but I cannot form them into a coherent statement to express the anger I felt against that facility. Nevertheless, I went and found Job agitated and pacing in a way no different than when he lived at home. He was alone in the dining room. He went from table to table adjusting the vinyl tablecloths. A broom was nearby. He took it and began to sweep the dining room. If he started to touch something that I thought he shouldn't, I quietly admonished him not to. Eventually the agitation subsided and I persuaded Job to let's go to his room. I helped him get undressed and get into bed. When I left him, he was sleeping.

The social worker at the psychiatric hospital had provided us with a list of nursing homes (it was decided that Job now needed "the next level of care"), and almost every day I had appointments to visit one. This was a very sobering and frustrating expe-

rience. I was to learn that Job's record of having been in a psychiatric hospital, as well as his record from the previous facility
were considered by other facilities in their decision to accept or
not accept him as a patient.

Some of the suggested places were simply unacceptable to
me. I had returned from a facility that I liked very much but
which would not accept Job. Before going to visit Job at the facility that he was in, I thought I would relax for a few minutes with
a cup of tea. I didn't get a chance to do that.

The nurse from the facility called with the message that the
one-on-one nurse hired to sit with Job was leaving at 3:00, and if
he should become combative and there was no one to stay with
him, they would call the police.

"Where will the police take him?" I asked.

"We don't know," was her reply.

With less than half an hour to reach the facility before three
o'clock, I went to care for Job. The next day we hired our own
one-on-one person to care for Job for twelve hours a day. They
bathed him, helped him with his meals, and got him ready for
bed before leaving in the evening.

Two days into the New Year, 2003, we received a call from
a nursing home that I had visited and liked saying that they
would accept Job as a resident in their long-term care unit. In
order not to have to pay further rent to the old facility, which did
nothing for him except provide a place for him to sleep, and three
meals a day, we moved Job into the accepting facility on January
3, 2003.

From the beginning I was apprehensive about Job's placement
in a non-Alzheimer's setting and could not understand why that
was done. It is apparent that my apprehension was justified when
after only three days of being in the new location, because of his
combative behavior, Job was admitted to the behavioral unit of a
medical hospital. Two weeks later, he is still there.

All employees in this unit are very kind and compassionate.
The unit administrators have assured me that they will do all
they can to get Job's behavior to where he can return to the nursing home. As much as possible, they will try to accomplish this
by using drugs that do not reduce him to a zombie-like state.

"And if that doesn't work, what are my options?" I ask. "Do

I have him committed to the State hospital for the insane?"

"You don't want to do that," I am told.

No, I don't want to do that, but I don't really know what to do, and there seems to be no one who can advise me in the matter.

I last visited him yesterday. He was sitting in a wheel chair. His head was bowed very low. He did not lift it up. His eyes were closed, and he rarely opened them. I fed what little lunch he would eat to him. He had difficulty sucking liquids up through a straw. I asked him questions and he mumbled incoherent answers. He knows his name because he always responded when I addressed him. I am not sure that he recognizes that I am with him.

My frustration demands that I be angry with someone. I am not angry with God for allowing this affliction to happen to Job. But I am angry and because I do not know to whom I should address my anger, it is all encompassing.

I blame the second level of stress that I've endured on institutions that claim to know how to treat Alzheimer's patients but in reality do not. It is like a game they play. They take an up front fee from you for placing your loved one with them, then they are incapable of providing the service you've paid them to perform.

Since all the trouble began with the places that I have placed him in, I have considered bringing Job home and resume caring for him (with twenty-four-seven help) myself. And the really sad, sad part of that is that it is no longer an option at all.

MARLIN PRESS
P.O. Box 2174
Warminster, PA 18974-2174

Name _____

Address _____

City _____ State _____ Zip _____

Number of copies @ $12.95 each	
Shipping and Handling $2.26 each	
Subtotal	
Sales tax (PA residents add 6%)	
TOTAL	

Make enclosed check payable to **Marlin Press**.

E-mail & credit card orders can be placed at www.Amazon.com.

For inquiries call: (804)874-2172.